Health Essentials

Acupressure

Jon Sandifer is an experienced teacher and practitioner of acupressure, shiatsu, macrobiotics, reflexology, oriental diagnosis, feng shui and 9 star ki. He was an early staff member of the East West Centre in London, a charity presenting the Japanese philosophy of macrobiotics, and has written many articles for newspapers and magazines. Five of his children were delivered with the assistance of acupressure

The Health Essentials Series

There is a growing number of people who find themselves attracted to holistic or alternative therapies and natural approaches to maintaining optimum health and vitality. The *Health Essentials* series is designed to help the newcomer by presenting high quality introductions to all the main complementary health subjects. Each book presents all the essential information on each therapy, explaining what it is, how it works and what it can do for the reader. Advice is also given, where possible, on how to begin using the therapy at home, together with comprehensive lists of courses and classes available worldwide.

The *Health Essentials* titles are all written by practising experts in their fields. Exceptionally clear and concise, each text is supported by attractive illustrations.

Series Medical Consultant
Dr John Cosh MD FRCP

In the same series
Acupuncture by Peter Mole
Alexander Technique by Richard Brennan
Aromatherapy by Christine Wildwood
Ayurveda by Scott Gerson
Chi Kung by James MacRitchie
Chinese Medicine by Tom Williams
Colour Therapy by Pauline Wills
Flower Remedies by Christine Wildwood
Herbal Medicine by Vicki Pitman
Homeopathy by Peter Adams
Iridology by John and Sheelagh Colton
Kinesiology by Ann Holdway
Massage by Stewart Mitchell
Natural Beauty by Sidra Shaukat
Reflexology by Inge Dougans with Suzanne Ellis
Self-Hypnosis by Elaine Sheehan
Shiatsu by Elaine Liechti
Spiritual Healing by Jack Angelo
Vitamin Guide by Hasnain Walji

ACUPRESSURE

For Health, Vitality and First Aid

JON SANDIFER

ELEMENT
Shaftesbury, Dorset · Rockport, Massachusetts
Melbourne, Victoria

First published in Great Britain in 1997 by
Element Books Limited
Shaftesbury, Dorset

Published in the USA in 1997 by
Element, Inc.
PO Box 830, Rockport, MA 01966

Published in Australia in 1997 by
Element Books
and distributed by Penguin Australia Ltd
487 Maroondah Highway, Ringwood, Victoria 3134

Accupress point illustrations by David Gifford
All other illustrations by David Woodroffe

Cover design by Slatter-Anderson
Page design by Roger Lightfoot
Typeset by WestKey Ltd, Falmouth, Cornwall
Printed and bound in Great Britain by Biddles Ltd, Guildford & King's Lynn

British Library Cataloguing in Publication
data available

Library of Congress Cataloging in Publication
data available

ISBN 1-85230-964-4

Note from the Publisher
Any information given in any book in the *Health Essentials* series is not
intended to be taken as a replacement for medical advice. Any person with a
condition requiring medical attention should consult a qualified medical
practitioner or suitable therapist.

Contents

List of Figures

For Michio and Aveline Kushi,
who first showed me how simple and practical
oriental healing can be

Acknowledgements

I AM DEEPLY GRATEFUL to those who got me started in this particular field and who answered my many questions with such patience. They include: Michio Kushi, Jacques de Langre and Mike Burns whose courses I attended in the 1970s.

Preface

FROM AN EARLY age, I have always enjoyed travel, adventure and independence. I was born and raised in Mombasa, Kenya, and came to school in England when I was nine years old. I had the benefit of an education in England and wonderful summer holidays in the Tropics. I attempted Mount Kilimanjaro when I was 14 and 16. At 17 years of age, I went to Spitzbergen with a group of school friends for six weeks. This inspired me to explore further and in September 1970 I began my travels which took me six years, passing through 52 countries working as I travelled and living for extended periods on a limited budget in Third World countries. During this time I was keen to remain fit, to maintain my health while in frequently vulnerable situations regarding the quality of food and water available. This led me to decide early on in my travels that when I eventually settled down I would like to practise some form of traditional healing that brought aspects of medicine back into the family and the community.

In 1977 I attended classes at the East West Centre in London, a charity presenting the Japanese philosophy of macrobiotics. The argument as I understood it was that as individuals we are responsible for our health and vitality through our lifestyle, our diet and our attitude. I learnt how to cook using natural foods and studied shiatsu massage, oriental diagnosis, Japanese folk remedies, yin/yang philosophy and acupressure.

Some of the acupressure that I studied was for the symptomatic relief of various aches and pains; a second application was a Japanese derivative known as dō-in, a wonderfully invigorating self-massage. Most classes and courses that I attended began with this and it is something I practise frequently to this day. In Chapter 5 I include a routine that you can practise yourself.

Having a toolkit of acupressure points up my sleeve over the years has helped immensely in my life to relieve pain or distress – not only for myself but for friends, clients, colleagues and family. I am convinced from my own personal experience that we can all use acupressure to relieve aches and pains and that at the same time it can help us to understand why the symptom has occurred and what we can do ourselves to prevent it from recurring.

I hope that you gain as much pleasure and interest from the subject as I have over the years. Please do feel free to contact me (through the publishers) with any feedback or questions and also if you wish to organize a workshop in your locality. Enjoy!

Jon Sandifer

1

What is Acupressure?

ORIENTAL HEALING HAS grown in popularity in the West in the past 30 years. This is largely due to the popularity of acupuncture which enjoyed a revival in China in the 1960s. There are currently several thousand practitioners of acupuncture in the West and many of these are doctors who have included acupuncture within their practice. Riding on the success and popularity of acupuncture are several other closely associated disciplines. These include Chinese herbal medicine, various forms of bodywork such as tai chi and chi kung, different forms of meditation and martial arts, and many folk remedies and massage systems that stem from the same underlying philosophy as acupuncture.

Acupressure is directly descended from acupuncture. It is relatively easy to learn and you can practise it on yourself. Unlike acupuncture where a practitioner inserts a needle you simply apply pressure usually with your thumb to the relevant acupressure point. To become an acupuncturist involves some three years of study, a deep knowledge of anatomy and physiology, completion of examination and membership of the relevant association. However, with acupressure, you simply need to know the different points to press to bring about relief. This book shows you these points, explains an invigorating acupressure routine that can help stimulate your energy, and gives you the theory behind acupressure and oriental medicine.

Acupressure is easy to learn and helps bring a certain level of healing back within our grasp. Throughout time, as human beings, we have brought comfort to others through touch. We constantly and instinctively rub and press parts of our body to relieve muscle aches and pains. Acupressure and its underlying philosophy explain in more detail how touch and pressure can bring about change. I was always impressed when I studied aikido that the instructor could bring relief in minutes from pain or minor injury simply by applying pressure to a few acupressure points, often not close to the site of the pain. Was it intuitive, was it logical, what did he do? Many of the answers to these questions will appear in the next two chapters.

ACUPRESSURE, DŌ-IN, SHIATSU

These three systems have one common thread – the oriental concept that the body is charged by 'chi' energy (pronounced 'chee') which travels along pathways on the surface of the body known as 'meridians'. Although chi has not been fully explained scientifically, it is believed in the West to be a form of electromagnetic charge. A meridian is not dissimilar to a river in many ways. It has a source, an end and various points along the way where things can accumulate. Along the meridians these points, known as 'acu' points in Chinese or 'tsubo' in Japanese, act as a form of pumping station allowing energy to focus before moving on to the next point on the meridian. Figure 1 shows the meridians and acu points. Applying pressure or inserting a needle into one of these points has the effect either of stimulating the energy where perhaps it has become stuck or stagnant, or of relieving pressure when chi has become overactive and needs dispersing. This will become clearer in chapter 2 when we look at diagnosis and at the kind of technique needed for each particular condition.

Acupressure is used to relieve symptoms by applying pressure to one or several acupressure points. The treatment can last anything from three to fifteen minutes and is confined to dealing with an acute, specific problem.

Dō-in is a Japanese interpretation of acupressure whose literal translation is 'the way with yourself'. The system is based upon acupuncture meridians which you stimulate or sedate yourself by pressing, stretching, pounding and rubbing the meridians and points on the surface of the skin. Unlike acupressure which deals with specific points, dō-in treats your entire body and all the meridians. It is really designed as a workout to benefit the individual by getting the chi moving. It is traditionally practised in

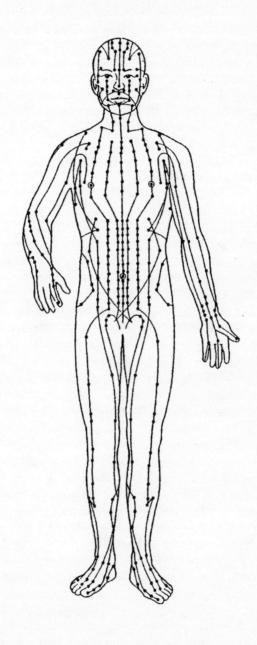

Figure 1 *A front view of the body showing acupuncture meridians and acu points*

the early hours of the day by martial artists and Buddhist monks. It is extremely beneficial and I encourage you to study the outline in chapter 6.

Shiatsu is another Japanese interpretation of acupressure – the literal translation being 'thumb or finger pressure'. Using the same understanding of meridians, points and chi, the shiatsu practitioner stretches your meridians or presses your acupressure points for you. The treatment works on most of the meridians, with additional stretches or focus on areas of acute stress. Treatment time is on average one hour. Unlike acupressure or dō-in you need to have a practitioner work on you.

THE ROOTS OF ORIENTAL MEDICINE

Most experts on oriental medicine acknowledge that the inspiration behind the development of acupuncture and its associated treatments lies with the Yellow Emperor who is believed to have lived between the years 2696 BC and 2598 BC. With the help of his students and philosophers, healers and teachers of the time, he began to develop a theory of human health. Much later, in perhaps the second or third century BC, much of the work was written down in the Chinese classic, the *Nei Ching*. This book forms the basis of oriental medicine and has been updated through the centuries. The influence of the *Nei Ching* can be found in Korea and in the sixth century AD the ideas also went to Japan where they were developed into the Japanese form of acupuncture, herbal medicine and massage. All the systems that evolve from the *Nei Ching* have one theme in common. This is that the body is governed by chi which travels through meridians and that along these meridians are some 400 acu points.

Different parts of China developed different approaches to the treatment of these points and meridians. For example, in the north of China, which was much colder, they preferred to treat the points using heat. This system of treatment is known as 'moxabustion'. Instead of the practitioner using a needle on the point they would apply heat close to the skin or in some cases actually on the skin at the point. Moxa itself comes from a herb (mugwort) which is commonly available in China as it is indeed in Europe. In moxabustion the moxa generally comes in three forms. The first is the loose herb itself which can be tightly compressed to form a small cone which then can be laid directly on the skin with the added protection of a small piece of onion skin or sometimes a sliver of ginger to protect the patient's skin. This cone is then ignited so that heat is transmitted down into the point. The cone is flicked off if it becomes too hot or painful. The second method is a cigar-shaped tube of mugwort which is ignited and held a quarter to half an inch (about 10 mm) away from the skin, rotated and the heat directed into the point. The third method is to use a moxa stick which looks similar to a joss stick. This is lit and having a finer end to it can be directed much closer to the point.

In the east of China where the climate was more humid and warm the local people were more prone to infection. It's in this part of the world that acupuncture developed. In the early days they used stone and bone needles, and later on steel ones. Historians also believe that these needles and primitive forms of surgery were used to lance infections.

In the west of China where it is more mountainous the use of herbs was developed. At the higher, colder altitudes plants become more concentrated and more focused in their effect. Most modern Western medicines owe their origins to plants and herbs and there is a growing interest in the West in the principles and the practice of Chinese herbal medicine.

In the south a slightly different form of acupuncture evolved known as the 'nine metal needle' system. This system uses a very small hammer which has nine needles on the head. Sometimes the handle of the hammer was made out of bone or turtle shell. The practitioner could then tap the head of this instrument over the point to bring energy to the surface or disperse energy that was blocked within the point. In Japan this system was known as the 'plum blossom'. The reason for this is that when you tap the points with the needles the chi and blood are drawn to the surface and the area becomes scarlet like plum blossom. It's not an unpleasant sensation and it's a little bit like the effect of a stinging nettle.

In central China the early forms of massage were developed and it is here really that we can trace the early origins of acupressure. Instead of needles or moxabustion the practitioner would use thumb or finger pressure on the points or meridians. Sometimes these acupressure points were used for diagnosis, other times for first aid and other times being incorporated into a fuller massage. As with most Chinese medicine, this form of massage travelled to Korea and on to Japan where it became the foundation of shiatsu.

USING ACUPRESSURE

Acupuncture has a deep and long-lasting effect. This means that practitioners need to be very well trained and absolutely clear about where they are going to place the needles and for what purpose. Herbal medicine too requires great skill because the effects are very immediate, deep and long lasting. Moxabustion in combination with acupuncture is again extremely powerful in its immediate effect and its long-term results. With the nine metal needle or plum blossom treatment the effects are immediate but last perhaps only three to four days. Likewise acupressure, and it is therefore a system that anyone can learn and practise on themselves knowing that they will not do themselves any harm.

The best way to learn acupressure is to practise applying pressure to some of the points on yourself so as to learn to experience the difference between the various points in terms of pain or any other sensation that you may feel. It's really only by practising on yourself initially can you begin to get a good sense of how these points can relate to different symptoms. For example, the 'stomach 36' point which is located just below the knee on the outside of the shin on both legs is a wonderful point to press if you're feeling physically tired or in need of a little boost. You can press this at work, or on a bus or if you're parked at the traffic lights. Always remember to breathe out as you apply the pressure and to breathe in as you release it. Repeat this process for six or seven breaths on each leg. When you locate the point correctly you may often feel something like a mild electric shock. (For a clear picture of where to find stomach 36 please look at page 43 in chapter 4.)

Perhaps the next time you have a headache instead of reaching for the paracetamol you could try a couple of the other points listed in chapter 4. If you're having some mild dental treatment and wish to control the pain yourself then ask your dentist to allow you to use acupressure on yourself, so long as you have a patient and understanding dentist who gives you plenty of time to breathe and is willing to cooperate. If your dentist likes to work quickly and has little patience then the success of your acupressure will be limited.

My children have always enjoyed a little acupressure from me for various aches and pains. If they trust you they can be very cooperative about the breathing process that is so essential, but only work with children if they want you to.

However, before going into more detail about specific acupressure points, we first turn to the principles behind acupressure and discover a little more about how it works.

2

The Principles of Acupressure

As EXPLAINED IN chapter 1, acupressure comes from the same stable as acupuncture, Chinese herbal medicine, moxabustion and massage. The feature that they all have in common is the same background understanding of the human body and its interaction with the external world. According to traditional Chinese philosophy, a human being is fuelled by four principle nutrients: food, fluid, air and chi.

Food is fundamental to our existence but we can live without it in extreme situations for quite some considerable time. It is not uncommon for individuals to fast for a day or two for health reasons and there are many cases of people who have lived some one hundred days without food, while continuing to take some fluid.

The second fuel of the body, fluid, is more important and we have a limited chance of survival without it. We could perhaps live five or six days without fluid but after this period we are risking dehydration and kidney failure.

The third fuel for our body is air and we are clinically dead if we do not receive this for three or four minutes.

The fourth fuel is chi, the Chinese expression for what we could call in English 'life force'. The Japanese call it 'ki', the Hindus 'prana' and the ancient Egyptians 'kaa'. We survive literally miniseconds without chi circulating in our system and so we should put it at the top of the list in connection with our survival. This energy, which is invisible, is regarded by the Chinese as the dynamic force that gives energy to our body, both in its development in embryo and in how we feel on a day-to-day basis.

If you were to look in a Chinese dictionary under the heading 'chi', you would find several pages of words for human emotions, as these are all understood to be manifestations of chi.

If we eat food that is fresh it has strong chi, having drawn this from the earth and rain that nurtured it. When we take water direct from a spring it is not only rich in oxygen but also rich in chi and this is what makes the water attractive and refreshing to drink. On the other hand we could draw water from a dark and stagnant pond and while essentially it is still water, it lacks the chi of a bright fresh mountain stream or spring. If we sit in a stuffy office or theatre we may find ourselves after several hours feeling tired, lethargic and out of touch with ourselves and our environment. If on the other hand we take a bracing walk through the woods or on a windswept beach we will feel charged by the chi. Similarly, we can feel the effect of the chi of a particular day. When it is bright and sunny we generally take on that mood ourselves. When the weather is cold and the nights are long and the prospect of spring is far away, our chi is depleted – which is why people crave the sunshine at that time of year and try to take a break to somewhere warm.

YIN AND YANG

There are two fundamental qualities of chi energy and it is their dynamic interaction that causes movement and change in ourselves and in nature. The chi which emanates from the earth and rises upward and outward in a diffusing spiral-like motion toward the heavens is known as the 'yin' force. On the other hand, chi energy that originates above and beyond us – in what the ancient people called heaven or the infinite – and that focuses and tightens its movement as it descends towards earth is known as the 'yang' force.

If we look at structures in nature we can see the interactions between these two forces in every facet of life. For example in the tree, its trunk, branches and leaves are seen as an expression of the upward yin force, whereas the roots bear all the hallmarks of the yang descending force. If you look at an oak tree which takes time to grow and is very hard and solid (yang) and compare it with a pine tree which is tall, fast growing with shallow roots and soft wood (yin), you can see that the oak is more yang than the pine tree. A carrot has a lot of root and activity below the surface and therefore although it has green leaves it has more yang force present in its development than yin. Compare this with a spring onion that has far more yin expression through its stem and vertical leaves and by comparison has very small and short roots.

In essence we could say that yin's nature is upward growth. As structures grow upward they become more diffused and often softer and they will then have a tendency to be lighter and cooler and ultimately begin to slow down. On the other hand, yang's nature is to grow downward and in that process to become more concentrated, therefore harder and often heavier. In this downward concentrated force the structures will often generate heat and speed up at the same time. Some other yin and yang qualities are listed in table 1.

The other principle of yin and yang to be aware of is that yin's nature at its extreme is to create its opposite, yang, and yang's nature at its extreme is to create its opposite, yin. If you were to plunge into an ice-cold bath (yin) it would not make you feel softer and more lazy or sleepy! In fact it would create the complete opposite, by making you feel alert, awake and extremely focused very fast. Similarly, a long hot bath (yang) would make you feel diffused and relaxed and slow you down.

When we look at the overall structure of the human being we can begin to see that with our vertical posture our brain and nervous system are positioned between heaven and earth, so acting as a kind of conductor for this yin and yang chi energy. The yin energy enters the body through the feet and the base of the spine rising up the body and exiting through the top of the head

Table 1 Yin and yang

Yin	Yang
cold	hot
passive	active
winter	summer
slow	fast
female	male
front	back
surface	deep
introvert	extrovert
mental	physical
chronic	acute

and the tips of the fingers. Conversely, yang energy enters the body through the fingertips and the top of the head, passing down the body and exiting through the base of the spine and the soles of the feet.

These channels of energy are the meridians. Those that carry the yin charge are found on the softer (yin) part of the body which is on the front. Yin meridians begin their path on the feet or in the armpits and rise upward terminating at the hands or the face but always keeping to the inner and the softer parts of the arms, legs, the torso and the face. Yang meridians are found at the beginning at the fingertips, at the side of the head or at the top of the head and descend toward the torso or the neck or the feet and keep themselves to the harder (yang) parts of the body as they make their journey downward.

We have twelve meridians, with six on the front of the body and six on the back, so that each has its equivalent or *partner*. (Table 3 on p 32 gives the partners.) One of the partners represents a yin direction and one a yang direction. (Appendix 2 explains which meridians are yang and which yin.) These twelve meridians also come in *pairs* – the same meridian on the left and right sides of the body. A final two meridians are to be located on the surface of the body but completely central at the front and the back passing over the spine and centrally down the front of the body. Ten of these meridians connect with internal organs as recognized in Western medicine. The last four meridians are connected with the overall circulation of the body's energy and not to actual organs.

One way of seeing our body from the oriental perspective would be to see it as an orchestra made up of many individual instruments. When one of these instruments is out of tune it affects the harmony of the whole orchestra and therefore the overall performance. The art of oriental diagnosis is to ascertain whether any of these instruments is lazy, slow, uninspired or sleepy (yin) or whether any of them are hyperactive, pushing, stuck or inflexible (yang). Having detected which instrument or organ needs attention the practitioner then begins either to stimulate (yang-ize) or to sedate (yin-ize) the organ or organs responsible. When attempting to treat yourself bear in mind also that symptoms that are fast, violent and painful are seen as more yang whereas those that come and go with a nagging kind of pain or come slowly are seen as more yin.

THE FIVE ELEMENT THEORY

Yin and yang provide us with a fundamental understanding of the cycle of energy in nature. Yin can represent the energy of dawn when we rise from the stillness of the night and begin the day's activity. This rising energy continues through the early hours and into our working activity and culminates at the midday point. At this time energy begins to slow down and in the afternoon the cycle continues towards the depth of night where energy becomes more yang. We can also look at this cycle in terms of the year where spring is connected with new beginnings (yin) and autumn is connected with the gathering in of the harvest (yang). From this understanding of the cycle of energy in nature the ancient Chinese developed a theory of five elements. I prefer to describe this as the 'five transformation' theory as it is connected with the way energy changes throughout the yin stage of the cycle culminating in creating the opposite yang stage of the cycle. Seeing it as a transformation cycle gives us the opportunity of observing the other stages as they merge from one into the other. These elements or transformational stages in nature also control our meridians and the related internal organs, with each being connected to different meridians and organs.

The five elements or stages are: wood, fire, soil or earth, metal and water. Each is covered in turn below. As you read through the five sections, make a mental note of symptoms or habits that you identify with as this will help you decide later (in chapters 4 and 5) which acupressure points or meridians you need to work on. Figure 2 shows the qualities and interactions of the five elements and the text below goes into these in more detail. Figure 2 also shows the meridians associated with each element. For more about the meridians see chapter 4.

The Elements

Wood

The literal translation of this stage of the cycle is indeed wood. However if you look more closely at the meaning it really represents the growth of young shoots, plants and trees and the rising energy of spring. I prefer to call this stage 'tree'. This element represents the forces of dawn or spring. It is the energy that gives

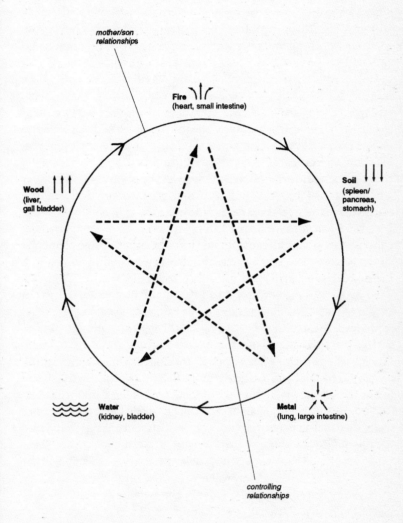

Figure 2 *The five elements, with their associated meridians and the relationships between the elements*

the impetus for new growth and change. The organs that are connected with this transformation are those of the liver and gall bladder.

When this element is strong in an individual they are very capable of initiating new ideas and new activities, they are very resourceful and good at beginning new projects, they find it easy to rise in the morning and are generally good humoured and flexible.

The liver is a producer of glycogen which provides energy for our muscles. If we are constantly feeling stiff in the joints, especially the knees and the elbows then this is usually related to an imbalance in the wood element. If we find it difficult to wake up in the morning and dislike the early hours then it is acknowledged that we have a wood imbalance. Many times the imbalance is due to overeating, especially the night before, or the intake of too much fatty food, alcohol or spice on the previous day. Instead of the liver resting through the night it has been overworking and this leaves us feeling tired and irritable the next day. Children are examples of people with very healthy livers as they are alert early and are generally happy in their waking process.

The springtime is when the element of wood is most active in a four seasons' climate and this can be noticed by the new sprouts of leaves, the new shoots coming up through the ground and the arrival of migrating birds. If we have become too yang or stuck during the winter we feel uncomfortable with this new rising energy. It is traditional in many cultures to help discharge the excesses of the preceding season by fasting and self-reflection (Lent) or by sauna (Scandinavia) or by traditional festivals and dancing which accompany the season in April or May. Activities that can also stimulate the tree energy in us include springclean-ing, dancing, singing and the use of new fresh vegetables that appear at this time of year. When we don't eliminate the heavy energy of winter we do not allow in the new fresh tree energy of spring and this can lead to stagnation in our health not only in the spring but also as we enter early summer.

To see how well your liver is at the moment you can apply pressure to the point called liver no 2 (see p 55). If you feel little or no pain your liver is in good shape but if the spot is painful to even a light touch then you may wish to take note of some of the preceding recommendations.

Fire

The rising energy of wood culminates in fire energy. Fire's nature is not only rising but also dispersing in a more horizontal direction. Whereas the tree nature was mostly vertical, fire energy is both upward and outward.

Fire is the element that controls the function of the small intestine and the heart, with the heart reflecting the movement of fire energy in its outward and inward pumping. The small intestine is connected through the Chinese understanding that it is the creator of the blood. Their argument is that we absorb our nutrients through the small intestine and this is regarded then as the starting place of the blood.

Fire as we observe it can have many different natures. If we make a fire with paper it will be all flame very quickly and die down to show us nothing. Fire made with coal or wood can be very bright and brilliant but at the same time maintain its heat and burn for several hours.

Diagnosing an imbalance in our fire nature can be done through observing how we are acting. An individual who is steady, warm, reliable and active will have strong fire energy, whereas someone whose behaviour is erratic has a weak or diminished fire nature. Ups and downs in our emotions, rapid swings in our mood and behaviour – one minute being enthusiastic and active and the next despondent and passive – all indicate imbalances in the fire element.

The two meridians called the 'heart governor' and 'triple heater' are controlled by fire. They are not so much connected with an organ but with our overall circulation and with our mental and spiritual state. Feeling the cold or uncomfortable in the heat is regarded as an imbalance of these systems, as is having a chaotic state of mind or a constantly changing direction in thoughts.

What is needed here to strengthen the fire energy is rhythm. One way of bringing this into our lives is to have a routine or to take up some activity which involves rhythm such as drumming. We can activate our fire energy by dancing or by singing or by combining the two as in some traditional tribal dancing ceremonies. Doing things in isolation or in the cold can dampen our fire nature, whereas socializing and being active with others can strengthen our fire nature. Many people who live in the colder parts of Northern Europe crave this fire element and rediscover it on their summer holidays to Florida or Spain. Fire is also central to the culture of all colder climates as the basis for cooking and industry. It is curious to think that despite the surrounding ice, Iceland is actually an island based on the underground fire that surfaces from time to time in the eruptions of lava and geysers.

Soil (or Earth)

At this stage of the five elements we begin to notice the settling quality of yang appearing. Another way of expressing soil (also known as 'earth') would be to say 'ashes', as they are created from the fire. Soil can also be represented as compost. Soil has a rich, supporting nature which is calm and stable.

This element controls the function of the spleen, pancreas and stomach. The spleen and pancreas in Chinese medicine are regarded as a storehouse of the body, with the pancreas dispensing blood sugar to the body. In a traditional Chinese community the storehouse and the storekeeper were central to the function and the future welfare of the community. Their job was not only to store the year's harvest but also to dispense it at a steady rate to the members of the community.

The season that this soil element represents is that of late summer and early autumn. If we were to look at the element in terms of the 24-hour cycle it would represent the afternoon. Often the afternoon is when people feel at their lowest in terms of energy and it is commonplace to stop work for five or ten minutes around 3 or 4 o'clock. People have tea or coffee or some kind of biscuit to raise their blood sugar level at this time. When our soil energy is strong we won't feel tired at that time of day and generally have steady energy throughout the 24-hour cycle.

The soil stage, as the gathering in and the calming down of the summer's energy, represents the completion of a cycle. When we translate this into our individual behaviour we can observe that if we are good at completing projects, letters, conversations and promises then our soil nature can be considered strong. If however we look around our home and notice areas of incompletion then we could argue our soil nature is weak. One way to strengthen our soil nature is to make a list of areas in our life that are not complete and begin to complete them. When this soil nature is strong then we can be very supportive, helpful and sympathetic towards others, but on the other hand when this area is weak we can become cynical and sceptical and display many symptoms of self-pity and apathy. Being in contact with the soil, either by taking long walks in the country or by gardening or by walking barefoot on the grass every day can help strengthen this element in all of us. We can also reduce the stress on the pancreas by eliminating sugar and other forms of highly refined carbohydrate from our diet as they demand so much energy from us just to assimilate the nutrients from them.

Metal

Taking this transformation cycle one stage further is metal, a concentrated version of soil. Whereas soil has a direct vertical downward energy, metal's nature is to contract from all directions. This could be regarded as the ultimate drawing in of energy toward the body. The metal energy controls the function of the lungs and large intestine and both of these organs relate to the drawing in of the external environment. The more active yang lung draws in and absorbs the more yin air, whereas the less active yin large intestine absorbs the more yang elements from our food. Although their primary function is to draw energy in these organs also eliminate residues and another way of seeing metal energy is as the more contracted version of soil which given time and pressure creates rock and mineral.

Given that metal's nature is so yang, then the imbalances that can be noted in our condition are also to do with an over-yang expression. This literally translates into becoming isolated, still, lacking in vitality, introspective and depressive. A way to counteract these qualities within us is to get more oxygen circulating in the body. Basic advice here is obviously not to smoke, to take regular exercise in the fresh air and to reestablish new patterns and ways of breathing. Tai chi, chi kung and yoga can be of immense value in this area. Making the effort to socialize and to be more animated in our expression and conversation will also help.

The metal stage also represents the final stages of autumn, the ultimate gathering of energy and of the harvest. This time, rather like the spring, is a good time to prepare ourselves mentally and physically for the next stage of transformation. Whereas in the spring we need to loosen up ('yin-ize') before the onset of warmer weather and the more social activities, we need time in the autumn to reflect and bring our energy to a focus and plan ahead for the long cold winter. I usually like to eat very simply for a ten-day period during the autumn to help clear out excess yin from my system to make the transition into deeper winter much more comfortable. This is also an ideal time to begin studies and most universities, schools and adult education classes start at this time of year.

Water

If we were to compress and to make more yang the metal element it would eventually melt and become liquid, like water. Water's nature can be seen as a floating stage where there is little or no activity.

This stage is clearly the deepness of night and the darker months of winter. Although disliked by many of us, it does provide an essential part of our lives as human beings. We all need the coolness of winter to internalize our energy, to rest, to learn and assimilate from the previous year and to prepare ourselves for the onset of spring. The night time and our sleep have much the same function for us. We all need sleep to repair, to regenerate, to reflect and to refresh ourselves for the next day's activities.

While they appear on the surface to be times of day or times of year that have no real value, they certainly do on a deeper level. If we stay awake all night then the next day we are tired and often poor in our creative skills. Similarly, if we work too hard during the winter time we can risk burning out by early spring and thereby miss out on the opportunities to re-create ourselves and redesign our future in the spring. It is not uncommon in our modern lifestyle that we put more strain on this element than any other one.

This element controls the function of the kidneys and the bladder, additionally the reproductive system and the adrenals. Tiredness and apathy are often connected with poor water energy and one of the simplest recommendations for this is sleep! Deep restful sleep can recharge the function of kidney, the use of warm foods and hot drinks and soups can also help give strength to the kidney. Keeping areas of the kidney meridian warm during the winter is also essential. It is very refreshing for our tree energy in the spring to walk barefoot on the grass but that same activity in midwinter could have the opposite effect on our water energy. We can see in winter that the trees have shed their leaves and that many animals have gone to sleep but this does not mean that they have died. Far from it: they are replenishing and conserving their energy at the same time.

The Relationships between the Elements

There are two relationships to be aware of in the five transformation theory. One, which we could call the 'mother/son relationship', is where the previous element is the 'mother' or the fuel of the next stage. In other words fire is the creator of ashes (soil), soil is the creator of rocks (metal), metal eventually dissolves and becomes liquid (water) which nourishes plant life (wood) which is the fuel of fire.

The second relationship is one of control. If one of the elements becomes overactive, then instead of fuelling the next stage in a healthy, helpful way it ignores the next stage and attacks the element opposite to it. For example the element wood is said to dig up the element earth, as the roots of a tree or a plant can break up the soil. Soil can dam the flow of water and water can extinguish fire. Fire can melt metal and metal can cut wood. There are ways of seeing this from a Western point of view. For example individuals with heart problems (fire imbalances) often have breathing difficulties or lung (metal) problems. It is also common that patients with kidney troubles or kidney failure (water) have often had pancreatic (soil) problems like diabetes. To take this whole area further I would encourage you to study the *Nei Ching*.

ORIENTAL DIAGNOSIS

Although this is an enormous subject in Chinese medicine, requiring a practitioner years of study, there are some basic principles that we can begin to appreciate and learn as we study and practise acupressure. A sound diagnosis forms the basis of any acupuncture, moxabustion or herbal treatment and it arises from many different observations that can be made on a patient. Further details are given in appendix 2.

Many of us practise oriental diagnosis in our daily lives without even knowing it. When we walk into a room and meet somebody for the first time we assess them, not in a clinical or intellectual way, not in a way that we have been taught from a textbook, but more intuitively. For example, are they happy, sad, tired, uneasy, distracted?

Similarly, oriental diagnosis is based on using all our faculties and the first of these is *sense*. Some would argue this is intuition, others that we can detect energy or aura from the person or that we simply pick up on whether the person is happy or sad, vibrant or depressed. Whatever the source of the information, sense is something we have all experienced. Think of the last time you entered a room and two individuals who were talking became silent and you could immediately sense they had been in the middle of a deep discussion or an argument. You can just feel it.

The second faculty used in oriental diagnosis is *sight*. When we look at an individual we can detect from their body language how they are feeling, what areas of the body they protect and what they are telling us from their different gestures. Often when they discuss their problems they could be pointing toward the area of pain or discomfort or sometimes protecting it. When somebody expresses themselves constantly with the upper part of the body, with their hands, their head and their eyes we can regard this as a fire expression. In Latin countries, which are naturally more fiery than colder Northern European countries, people use their head, eyes and hands continuously in their communication. A Northern European may see this sort of behaviour as fire imbalance.

Sight is also used to diagnose in more detail. For example the skin is studied – its colour, its blemishes, scars or moles. The meridians can be studied. The hair and the face are studied and lines or discoloration are correlated to the major internal organs. For example if the hair is bright, strong and full of vitality this indicates that the intestines are also healthy. Conversely, hair that is limp and weak is one of the first signs of poor absorption and poor digestion. The peripheral parts of the body such as the fingers and toes can also be studied. Clearly defined cuticles show an individual who has a steady digestion and is not chaotic in their eating habits. Strong but flexible nails indicate a good rounded diet. If the colour resumes very quickly to a nail after it has been pressed this is a sign that the blood is in good shape, whereas if the nail remains white for up to half a minute this shows that the person is anaemic. Discoloration in different parts of the eyes can indicate stagnation in corresponding areas of the body. Sensitivity to light is usually a sign of a liver imbalance. The study of the tongue is also of major importance in oriental medicine.

Diagnosis is also made by *listening*. This is not diagnosing a person by questioning them about their habits and how they feel but more listening to the underlying tone of their voice. This kind of diagnosis relates back to the previous section on the five element theory. If an individual has an erratic voice, constantly stops and starts while they speak or changes the tack of their conversation that is a sign of a fire imbalance. Since one of the strengths of the soil element is completion then, when an individual speaks and there is incompletion in their communication, that is a sign of a soil imbalance. This could be sentences that trail off to an incomplete conclusion or a 'sighing' quality, where each sentence trails off into a kind of sigh. A wood imbalance is indicated by a voice that is abrupt and by curtness of expression or someone who sounds as if they are shouting. With a metal imbalance the voice lacks power, variety and vitality with the person coming across as if they are groaning. With a water imbalance it sounds as if the person is weeping. If you listen carefully to the voice it sounds as if the person is on the edge of tears, their voice having a soft almost watery quality to it. Rather like the flow of a river their conversation may ramble and appear to a certain extent inconclusive.

Another method of diagnosis that was not only practised in China but also in India by 'Ayurvedic' doctors, is diagnosis by *smell*. All of us have an individual odour that is emanating from us and if the smell is violent then it is an indication of some kind of imbalance. Try and remember the last time you visited somebody who was ill in bed and you may recall there was a distinct smell in the room when you entered. If you bring someone a cup of tea in the morning who has had a fever in the night then you can smell a strong odour in the room and traditionally all hospitals insisted on fresh air to help in the healing process. With skill and practice these smells can be related back to the organ involved and even what kind of food the person was eating to create that kind of imbalance.

Another method of diagnosis is through *touch*. Again diagnosis through touch is something we frequently do when we meet an individual. What does their handshake tell you? Is it cold, does it lack any real power? If so then we may be left with the impression that their condition is more yin. If however their grip is firm, their palm is dry and warm then this is an indication that their condition is more yang. An excessively yang person will squeeze your hand so hard that you are unlikely to forget the event in a hurry! The most accurate and complete method of diagnosis favoured by acupuncturists is the examination of the pulses located on the inside edge of both wrists. There are three points on each wrist, each of which can be examined at two levels. This gives a total of twelve pulses corresponding to the six main pairs of meridians. There are twenty-eight different pulses in total and it requires years of study to be able to use them all.

Diagnosis is also made by observing *habits and behaviour*. For example, somebody with a fire imbalance would tend to be more scattered in their approach to taking on a task – they would begin with great enthusiasm and then become either despondent or lethargic. We all know individuals like this who are blowing hot and cold most of the time. Similarly, they change tack in their conversation or continually change their mind. They frequently suggest one thing and do the opposite. A soil imbalance is reflected in a somewhat apathetic and despondent approach to life or difficulty in completing projects or courses of action. Someone with a metal imbalance prefers to do things alone, quietly, perhaps in great detail, and has real difficulty in expressing their feelings, leaving you with the impression that they have no vitality. Someone with a water imbalance appears shy and retiring, dithery and unable to make a commitment. Someone with a wood imbalance comes across as insensitive to their immediate environment or to their neighbours, and possibly intimidating or boisterous. Their expression is loud and enthusiastic, and sometimes rigid or stubborn.

Having looked at some of the theory behind acupressure, we now look at how acupressure works in practice.

3

How Does it Work?

ACUPUNCTURE AND ACUPRESSURE have been practised in the Far East for over five thousand years. As explained, what the systems have in common is an understanding that the body is governed by the flow of chi energy. Any distraction in the flow of this chi energy or any upset to the internal organs will consequently upset the flow of chi. It is therefore the realignment of chi through the use of needles, pressure or herbs that forms the basis of Chinese medicine. How this works is a growing area of investigation in the West. Like the electromagnetic energy in our nervous system, chi is vibrational and invisible and the question of how it works is open to discussion. However, there are some theories which have been developed in the past 30 years, mainly to do with acupressure's pain-relieving abilities.

WESTERN IDEAS

Endorphin – The Body's Natural Painkiller

Our body produces its own painkiller known as endorphin. This is a protein molecule which is created and stored by our 'endocrine system' (our glands). The release of the endorphin molecule is controlled by our nervous system. Our nervous system relies on messages from nerves and nerves react to external stimulation through the senses. In response to certain external stimuli the nervous system causes the endocrine system to release endorphin. Pressure on the acu points has a similar effect and this may well be a modern explanation of the success of acupressure in controlling pain.

The 'Gate Control' Theory of Pain

In 1965 Ronald Melzach, a Professor of Psychology at McGill University in Canada, presented a theory of how pain arises and its possible treatment. Through research he discovered that if the nerve fibres within the nervous system had their impulse distracted it affected how the nervous system dealt with receiving these messages. Within the bundles of nerves are individual fibres each with different tasks. Some of these fibres receive and transmit information, others carry the sensation of pain, others react to the external world whilst others react to the internal world of the body. What Ronald Melzach discovered was that if the fibres that carry impulses relating to touch, pain, temperature and so on could be stimulated selectively this in turn blocked the impulses in the fibres that carried the sensation of pain. Acupuncture and acupressure have both been found to stimulate the nerve fibres associated with touch and pressure and may now account for the anaesthetic qualities which are associated with them.

TOWARDS A MORE HOLISTIC UNDERSTANDING

Pain control however is not the only function of acupressure and, indeed, removing pain without looking at its causes can be dangerous. So how does acupressure work on a more general level? Frequently you find yourself fumbling around in the dark attempting to answer this question in the scientific, logical or technical way that is expected in the kind of culture in which we live. It must be appreciated that oriental and Indian medicine and traditional folk remedies have been widely practised and used by human beings for thousands of years. It is only in the past century or so that they have become marginalized. Since you are already becoming familiar with yin and yang we could look at the question from that perspective.

Subtle methods of healing that involve touch, plants, herbs, flowers, smells, needles and massage really depend on an understanding of the body in a vibrational way (yin). A wider perspective on understanding the human being and connecting it with the environment, nutrition, activity and so on can be regarded as seeing a bigger more 'holistic' picture (yin). We are now living in a much more active, focused, detailed culture (yang) and this is reflected in all aspects of our lives.

While we all enjoy the benefits of this more yang phase in human development it can also cause us to see things in such minute detail that we fail to see the big picture. It is often easier for us to focus on one area of a human being and fail to connect it with any other dimension. This is very clear when you enter any modern hospital in the Western world and are greeted by a list of departments where they specialize either in particular ailments or parts of the body. The more we become an expert in one specific area the less we are going to notice the larger picture. The direction we have taken these last one hundred years in Western medicine is a more yang-focused approach to seeing the human being. The way this is expressed now is in the diagnosis and study of blood, our bones, cells, genetics and DNA.

The further we pursue this route, which I am sure we must, the more likely it is that we will reach the extreme expression of it which will mean there is no further we can go. Once we get to this point, probably in the next 20 years, there will be a natural tendency to begin to take a wider view of the human being once more.

So many so-called 'holistic healing' methods are essentially working with the human being on a vibrational level. Seeing the interrelatedness of symptoms is very yin. All the small components that we study now in such detail are microcosms of the whole. The future definitely lies with vibrational healing and the growing interest in the past 20 years only serves to support this.

PRACTICAL APPLICATION

The unique quality of acupressure is that you are diagnosing and treating yourself. You are not using any inanimate instruments but using your own pressure and your own chi to bring about changes.

What is so closely knitted to the circulation of chi is our breath and it is important to remember that you apply pressure always on the out-breath. When you breathe in, you are activating your system not only with oxygen but also with chi and as you breathe out you eliminate excess chi from the system as well as waste from the breath. As we breathe out we are able to relax more deeply and to feel the benefit of the pressure occurring at the time.

It is not uncommon that in minor injuries you do the exact opposite. For instance if you cut or burn yourself the immediate reaction is to breathe in and often hold the breath. This can make the situation a little more painful and leave you more stressed as a result. The real key to success with acupressure is to be able to breathe out as you apply the pressure.

As you apply the pressure, do not jab into the point. Approach it slowly and go down to a level at which you feel a certain resistance and on the border line with what feels painful. If you press a point that is painful, do not go beyond the pain barrier as this will often have an opposite effect to the one you are trying to achieve. When the point is extremely tender, my advice is to approach it slowly and gently (on the out-breath), and apply the pressure in a spiral motion. If you do this you will notice how the point begins to open up. Relax the pressure as you breathe in and then repeat the pressure as you breathe out, taking the full breath to go to that point of resistance. If you repeat this process six to eight times you will begin to notice that the area softens and allows you deeper access.

The image I often have in my mind when I apply pressure is that of pressing down through layer upon layer until I find some solid ground. It is not dissimilar to walking on mud, where initially you sink but after a short while you meet with some resistance and then although you are still descending you find somewhere where your feet settle on terra firma. It is not always possible to achieve this if you stab at the points and this is why it is essential to work slowly and carefully.

EXAMPLES

Here are four points that you can practise on yourself as a way to get you started with acupressure. These are commonly used acu points that are easy to locate. Please use the advice from the previous section in relation to pressure and technique. Do not forget to do both hands or legs and attempt each side of the body at least six times. The points are illustrated in the next chapter.

Large Intestine 4

In Chinese this point is called the 'great eliminator' and it is a good point for tonifying the digestive system, both in cases of constipation and on a daily basis to strengthen our digestion. The point is located midway between the thumb and the forefinger in the fleshy part very close to where the bones meet high up in the valley.

Bring your opposite hand across to this area. Breathe in and then, as you breathe out, slowly begin to apply the pressure until you feel resistance or pain. Hold the point for the rest of the out-breath and as you breathe in begin to release the pressure for the rest of the in-breath.

This should be repeated five times, then move to the other hand.

Heart Governor 6

This is an excellent point for calming the mind if you are stressed or suffering any shock.

To locate this point look on the inside of your wrist and bring your opposite thumb across until you are midway along the wrist close up in the small valley next to the wrist. With the outside edge of your thumb you will feel the bones on your wrist and you apply the pressure between the tendons on the inside of your wrist.

Breathe in and as you breathe out apply the pressure until you feel resistance or pain. Hold the pressure for the complete out-breath – it is important not to let go of the point.

Repeat the process five more times and then move to the other side.

Kidney 1

In Chinese this point is called 'bubbling spring'.

This is a very deep point that can be found on the sole of your foot in a valley between the hard skin located below your big toe and the other area of hard skin on the ball of the foot under your four toes. Because this point is deep you need to press it firmly and repeat the process at least ten times. You may find that the point becomes more responsive as you work on it.

The kidneys are the source of our vitality and this point is especially good for fatigue, lethargy, for grounding energy and combating an over-intellectual lifestyle.

Stomach 36

The Chinese for this could be translated as the '3 mile point' and it is an excellent point for giving your body a physical boost when you need the extra reserves for physical activity or for staying up later at night. The idea is that if you stimulate this point well you will have the energy to go an extra 3 miles (or at least the Chinese equivalent)!

This point is found along the stomach meridian which is located on the outside of your shinbone just below your knee. An easy way to locate it is to place the palm of your left hand over your left kneecap. Stomach 36 is then directly below the pad of your middle finger. At this point bring over your right hand and begin to apply pressure with your right thumb.

It is good advice to wiggle your thumb around while the pressure is on until you find the point. You will know when you find it as it will give you a sensation a little bit like a mild electric shock or when you catch a nerve in the elbow region.

Work with this point five or six times and repeat this process on the other side.

What I initially learnt years ago about acupressure was that I could start to be responsible for many of the so-called accidents that I had. When you look back objectively at what you were doing, what kind of stimulation you received, what condition your mind and body were in, you can start to see that these accidents were in fact the sort of stimulation that you needed at the time.

For example, burning yourself is an extremely yang stimulation and areas that we burn on our hands and our wrists often relate to our circulation and to our breathing.

Perhaps you have woken up tired and sluggish after a late night when you ate shortly before going to bed, or you may have had more alcohol than you usually do, and as a consequence your liver is feeling sleepy in the morning. That always manifests as feeling irritable and impatient and in your rush to get yourself organized you may have stubbed your big toe very hard on a chair or on the door. If you check on the meridian chart you will discover that this is where your liver meridian begins.

We all have a wonderful opportunity to reflect on the stimuli that we have given ourselves or that we receive from our external environment.

GUIDELINES FOR USING ACUPRESSURE

With your new unbridled enthusiasm to try out some of these acupressure points, please let me remind you that it is important in the initial stages that you practise them on yourself. If, however you do choose to try these points on family or friends, here are guidelines as to when *not* to use acupressure.

1 Do not apply acupressure to an area where there is broken skin.
2 Do not apply acupressure to areas of skin that are infected.
3 Please avoid applying any pressure to areas of the body that may have varicose veins.
4 I would avoid using acupressure in cases of a high fever.
5 Always avoid trying a point on someone that you have not applied to yourself. This is only commonsense as you will not know what it feels like or what the effect is like.
6 The most obvious time when not to give someone acupressure is when they do not want you to. In our enthusiasm to help we should not forget to respect other people's wishes.

4

First Aid

THIS CHAPTER IS designed to give you a quick and easy access to acupressure points that can help relieve a variety of symptoms. A majority of these points you can access yourself. However, many of the bladder meridian points (*see* p 50–1) will need the help of a friend. It is important to stress that if you suspect that you have a chronic medical problem that the acupressure has not relieved, you should seek the advice of a competent medical practitioner. The information here is designed to bring you relief from a symptom and it is not intended as a substitute for any treatment that has been prescribed by your doctor.

The measurements I have used for locating the points are based on the traditional acupuncturist's measurement of the 'cun'. When measuring the points it is important to remember that they are based on the *receiver's* fingers or thumbs. The three basic measurements that are used in acupressure/acupuncture are as follows:

- *One cun* – one thumb's width
- *One and a half cun* – two fingers' width
- *Three cun* – four fingers' width

However, to make this book easy and accessible, I have not used the term 'cun', but have instead referred to a thumb's, two fingers' or four fingers' width.

For some of the symptoms listed, I have given a variety of points for acupressure and it is better to try one pair at a time. (By a pair I am referring to the one point, but on both sides of the body.) With practice and experience you may derive benefit from using one or two pairs. Initially, the less you do, with the more focus and intention, the more likely you are to see a result. If you go into the process sceptically or with little positive focus or vitality then you are more likely to have a weaker result.

Always remember never to press any of these points causing any kind of pain as this will not allow the energy in the point and the meridian to move. If you press too hard you are really distracting the chi in the point.

Always remember to breathe from your belly, to breathe out whenever you apply the pressure, and as you breathe in to relax the pressure.

Remember also, that the meridians (apart from those on the conception and governing vessel meridians, *see* p 66 and pp 63-4) each have partners (*see* table 3, p 32) and you must apply pressure to the partner meridian as well as to both sides of the body.

I also find it very helpful to focus clearly and intentionally on what you are trying to achieve. If you are attempting to release pain from a symptom then as you apply the pressure and breathe out imagine the symptom dispersing, becoming softer and leaving you in a more restful state.

You may find it useful to be aware of when there is more energy in each meridian. There is a peak time of day when there is far more focus for two hours in each of the 12 meridians, making the associated organ far more receptive to the work that you are doing. This cycle of twelve meridians multiplied by two hours gives us a full 24-hour cycle, as shown in table 2. It may be very inconvenient to get yourself up between 1 and 3am to stimulate your liver, but it is worth noting that it is often by being overactive, eating or

Table 2 The 24-hour cycle and the meridians

Stomach	7am–9am
Spleen/pancreas	9am–11am
Heart	11am–1pm
Small intestine	1pm–3pm
Bladder	3pm–5pm
Kidneys	5pm–7pm
Heart governor	7pm–9pm
Triple heater	9pm–11pm
Gall bladder	11pm–1am
Liver	1am–3am
Lungs	3am–5am
Colon	5am–7am

drinking alcohol at this time that we damage the energy of the liver.

Some of the acupressure points work primarily because they are on a meridian that is connected to the organ that is creating the imbalance. However, some of the points work because they are located in an area which is close to the offending symptom; others because the point is on a pathway where meridians connect to the symptom. For example, the acupressure points that can bring relief for toothache are beneficial because the meridian passes close to the jaw where the roots of the teeth are. Another example is the location of points on the shoulders which can be associated with digestive disorders as the meridians of the large intestine, small intestine and gall bladder pass through this region.

The sections below and the diagrams should help you start to locate the different meridians and acu points. The different symptoms and their treatment are given at the end of the chapter.

THE MERIDIANS

Table 3 lists the meridians and the associated acu points. The meridian partners are bracketed together. Figure 2 p 13 shows which elements the meridians are associated with.

Table 3 The meridians and their acu points

Name of meridian	Abbreviation	Number of acu points
Lung	LU	11
Large intestine	LI	20
Spleen/pancreas	S/P	21
Stomach	ST	45
Heart	HT	9
Small intestine	SI	19
Bladder	BL	67
Kidney	KD	27
Liver	LV	14
Gall bladder	GB	44
Heart governor	HG	9
Triple heater	TH	23
Governing vessel	GV	28
Conception vessel	CV	24
14 meridians		**361 acu points**

SYMPTOMS AND THEIR TREATMENT

Acidity	BL21
Altitude sickness	S/P9
Amnesia	HT7
Anxiety	HT3
Asthma	LV1 BL13 S/P9 CV17
Bad breath	HG8
Bedwetting	LV3
Blurred vision	BL4 BL5
Breast pain	CV17
Bronchitis	BL13 LU1 LV14
Chest pain	HT1
Colds	LU7
Conjunctivitis	GB1 ST19
Constipation	S/P12 ST25 GV20
Coughing	LU5 HG3
Coughing, chronic	LU9
Cystitis	S/P6 LV8 BL18 BL27 BL28
Depression	CV17 LU11 HT9 SI1
Diabetes	CV12 BL20
Diarrhoea	ST25 CV6
Dizziness	ST8 BL62
Dry skin	SI3
Earache	TH20 TH17 KD6 GB8 SI18
Elbow pain	SI8 TH5 HT3
Eye disorders	BL18 GB44
Fatigue	ST36 CV4 HG8 CV6 TH20
Fever	LG11
Flatulence	CV8 KD14
Fluid retention	KD3
Frozen shoulder	SI10 BL13 TH17 GB21
Gall stones	BL18 BL19 BL20 GB24
Gout	KD3

Haemorrhoids	GV20 BL57
Hangover	S/P6
Headache	GB21 BL10 LI4 LI11 SI1 LV1
Hepatitis	LV14
Hiccoughs	TH17 ST36
Hoarseness	LI18
Hypertension	KD2 BL15 BL23 GV24
Hyperventilation	ST41 HG6 LU5
Impotence	BL22 BL23 CV4 CV7
Incontinence of urine	S/P10
Influenza	GV16 TH5
Insect bites	BL66
Insomnia	LU9 S/P6 ST45
Irritability	LV3 HT7
Jaundice	BL18 BL19 CV14
Kidney disorders	ST27 KD1
Kidney fever	BL22
Kidneystones	GB25
Labour	BL60 BL67
Lactation problems	SI1 ST25
Laryngitis	TH1
Liver disorders	BL18 LV14
Lower back pain	BL23 BL58
Lumbago	BL27
Lung disorders	BL13
Mental fatigue	LI11
Mental tension	S/P1 KD1 GB18 GB44
Migraine	BL7 GB12 GB20
Morning sickness	CV12 ST36
Muscle disorders	BL18
Nasal congestion	LI20 ST3
Nausea	ST36 CV12
Neck pain	BL7 ST5
Night sweats	BL15 BL17
Nose bleeds	HG8 LI20

Pain	LI4 HG6 S/P6
Panic attacks	HG6
Phlegm on chest	LU1
Premenstrual tension	LU8 S/P6
Puffy eyes	GB20
Rheumatism	BL15 LI15
Sciatica	BL27 BL28 BL36 BL57
Shock	LU7 HG6 HG9 GV26
Shoulder stiffness	SI11
Sinus congestion	GV16 BL20
Sneezing	LU7
Sore throat	LI1 LU5 LU11 KD6
Sprain	
neck	BL10
shoulder	GB21
elbow	LI11
wrist	SI4 and 5
knee	ST35
ankle	BL60
Stomach spasms	CV12 GB24
Stress	HT7 HG8 GB34
Stuffy nose	BL10
Tinnitus	ST19 HT3
Tired eyes	BL1 ST36 LI14
Tongue ulcers	HT5
Toothache	LI4
upper	LI20
lower	ST6 ST7 ST42
Travel sickness	HG6 ST36 LV2
Twitch of the eyelid	ST1 ST2
Vertigo	BL18
Vomiting	BL23 CV17 CV10 ST36 S/P4
Water retention	LV13
Wrist pain	TH4 SI4

Lung Meridian (LU)

LU1

Between the first and second ribs, below the middle of the collarbone.

LU5

On the inside edge of the elbow, on the thumb side of the arm.

LU7

Above the wrist crease, on the thumb side of the arm.

LU8

In the hollow above the wristbone, on the thumb side of the arm.

LU9

On the wrist crease, in the hollow below the thumb.

LU11

Where the bottom of the nail touches the inside edge of the thumb.

Large Intestine Meridian (LI)

LI4

High up in the valley formed by the thumb and forefinger.

LI11

Make a 90 degree angle with the forearm and upper arm. The point is at the end of the crease that forms.

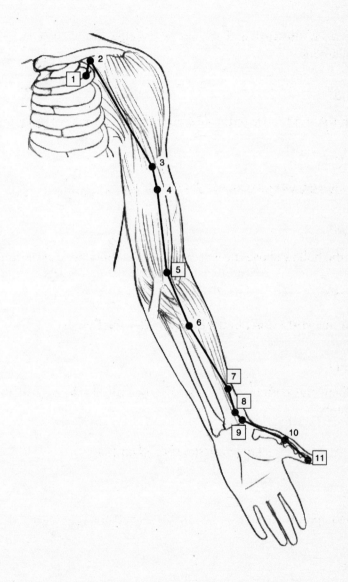

Figure 3   Lung meridian (LU)

LI14

On the outside edge of the upper arm, midway between the elbow and shoulder.

LI15

In the hollow on the outside edge of the shoulderbone.

LI18

On the outside edge of the neck and level with the Adam's apple in men.

LI20

In the hollow where the nostril meets the cheeks.

Spleen/Pancreas Meridian (S/P)

S/P4

In the depression beside the base of the first metatarsal bone, where the upper and lower part of the foot join.

S/P6

Three fingers' width above the anklebone, close to the shinbone.

S/P9

In the hollow, below the knee, close to the tibia.

S/P10

Three fingers' width above the kneecap, on the bulge of the muscle.

S/P12

In the groove, midway between the groin and the hipbone.

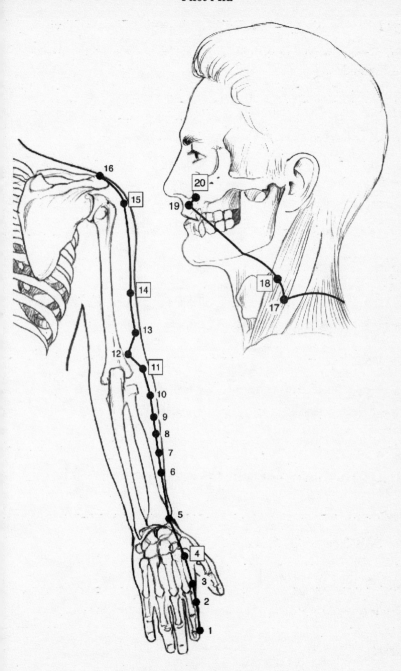

Figure 4 Large intestine meridian (LI)

Stomach Meridian (ST)

ST1

Between the lower eyelid and the eye socket.

ST2

Below ST1, on the bone of the eye socket.

ST3

Directly below the eye, under the cheekbone.

ST5

On the lower jaw, in the depression formed when the jaw muscle is clenched.

ST6

Above the corner of the jaw, one thumb's width forward toward the nose.

ST7

Where the upper and lower jaw meet, in the hollow when the muscles are relaxed.

ST8

On the edge of the forehead above ST7, just outside the hairline by half a thumb's width.

ST19

Measure two thumbs' width out from the navel, then go directly up until you meet the ribs.

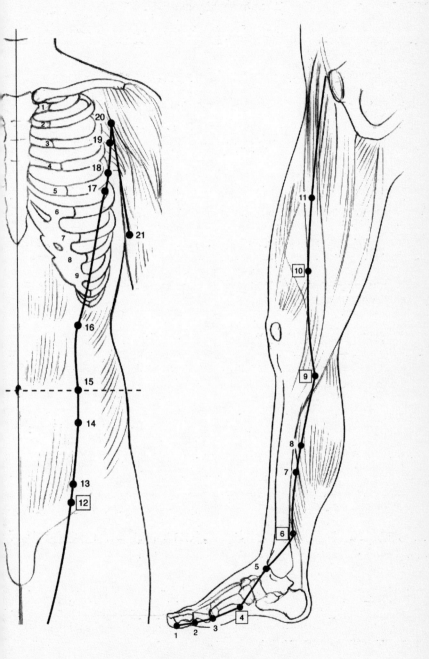

Figure 5 Spleen/pancreas meridian (S/P)

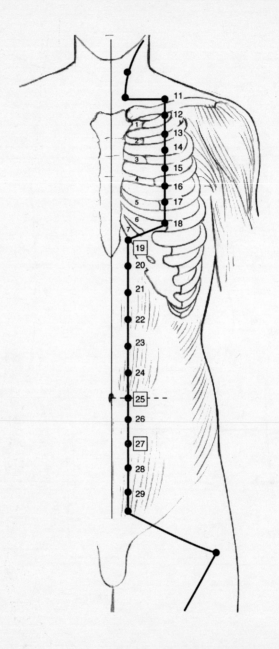

Figure 6   Stomach meridian (ST) (above and opposite)

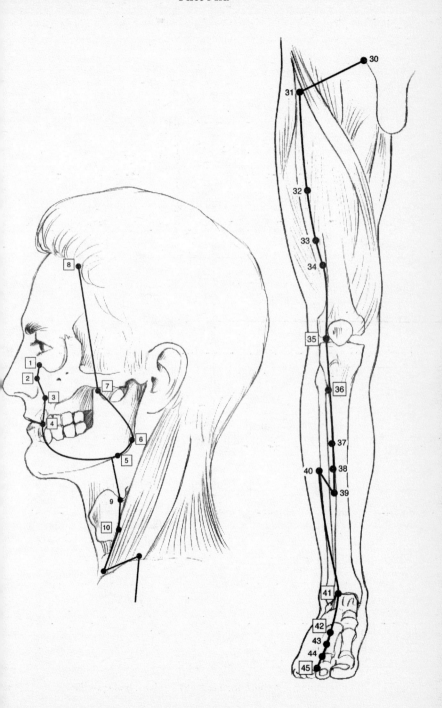

ST25

Two thumbs' width, either side of the navel.

ST27

Two thumbs' width either side of the navel and then measure two thumbs' width below.

ST35

Flex the knee and the point is in the depression below the kneecap.

ST36

In the hollow outside the shinbone, three fingers' width below the kneecap.

ST41

Flex the foot and the point is in the hollow where the foot meets the shinbone.

ST42

At the highest point of the foot, directly below ST41 and in line with the second and third toes.

ST45

On the outside edge of the second toe where the nail touches the flesh.

Heart Meridian (HT)

HT1

In the centre of the armpit.

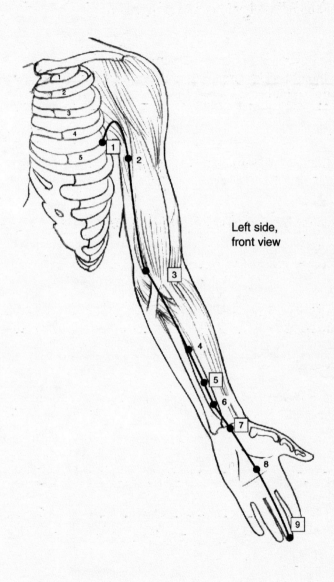

Left side,
front view

Figure 7   Heart meridian (HT)

HT3

With the elbow bent, it can be found just inside the elbow, against the bone.

HT5

With the palm facing upwards, the point is on the inside edge of the wrist, one thumb's width above the crease in the wrist.

HT7

On the wrist crease in the hollow below the little finger.

HT9

Inside of the little finger at the corner of the nail at its base.

Small Intestine Meridian (SI)

SI1

On the outside edge of the little finger, where the back of the nail touches the flesh.

SI3

On the crease formed by making a fist on the edge of the hand below the little finger.

SI4

In the hollow on the hand in the space between the hand and the arm.

SI5

On the outside edge of the hand, in the space between the hand and the arm.

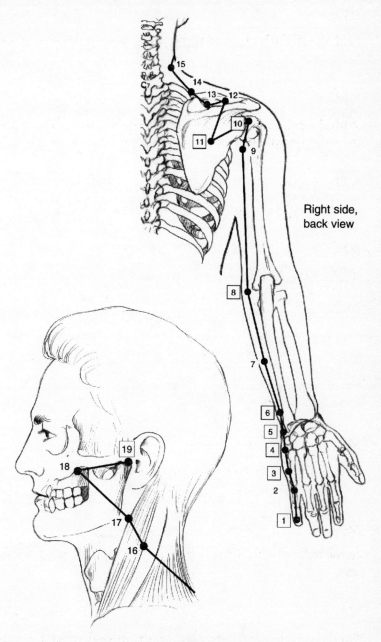

Right side,
back view

Figure 8   Small intestine meridian (SI)

SI6

Just behind the bony ridge of the wristbone, in the depression.

SI8

In the hollow behind the elbow on the outside of the arm.

SI10

On the outside edge of the shoulderblade, directly below the 'spine' of the shoulderblade.

SI11

Two-thirds up the ribcage in the middle of the shoulderblade.

SI19

In the depression between the jaw joint and the middle part of the ear.

Bladder Meridian (BL)

BL1

In the corner of the eye.

BL4, 5, 6, 7

Draw an imaginary line over the centre of the head from the nose to the base of the skull. The points are one thumb's width parallel to this channel – with BL4 just inside the hairline.

BL10

Below base of skull, one thumb's width out from the middle of the neck.

BL13

Level with the third thoracic vertebra a distance of one thumb's width away from the spine.

BL15

Level with the fifth thoracic vertebra.

BL17

Level with the seventh thoracic vertebra.

BL18

Level with the lower border of the ninth thoracic vertebra.

BL19

Level with the tenth thoracic vertebra.

BL20

Level with the eleventh thoracic vertebra.

BL21

Level with the twelfth thoracic vertebra.

BL22

Level with the lower portion of the first lumbar vertebra.

BL23

Level with the space between the second and third lumbar vertebrae.

BL27

At the point of the first depression in the sacrum.

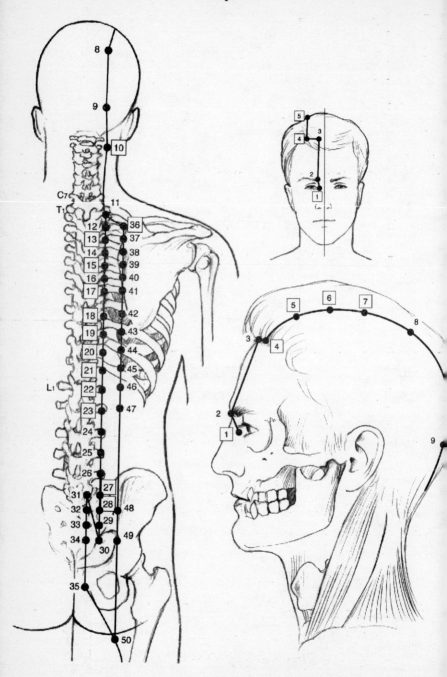

Figure 9   Bladder meridian (BL) (above and opposite)

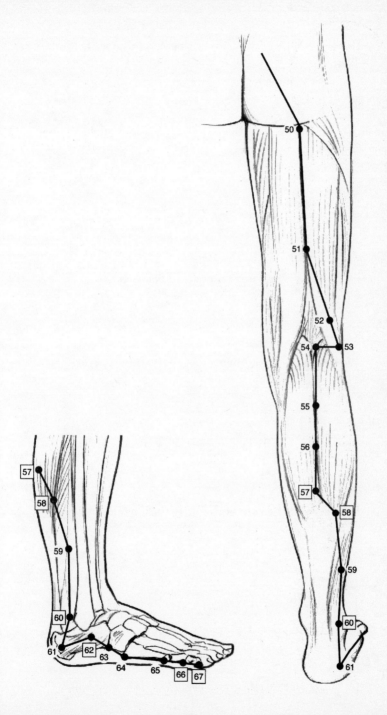

BL28

At the third depression in the sacrum, in line with the bladder meridian.

BL36

Just inside the shoulderblade, in line with the top of the shoulder-blade.

BL57

In the hollow in the centre of the calf muscle.

BL58

Directly above BL60, further out and below BL57 on the edge of the muscle.

BL60

On the outside of the ankle, between the ankle and Achilles tendon.

BL62

In the hollow directly below the anklebone.

BL66

In the hollow at the base of the little toe, on the edge of the foot.

BL67

On the outside edge of the little toe, at the base of the nail.

Kidney Meridian (KD)

KD1

In the valley in the ball of the foot. This is a deep point.

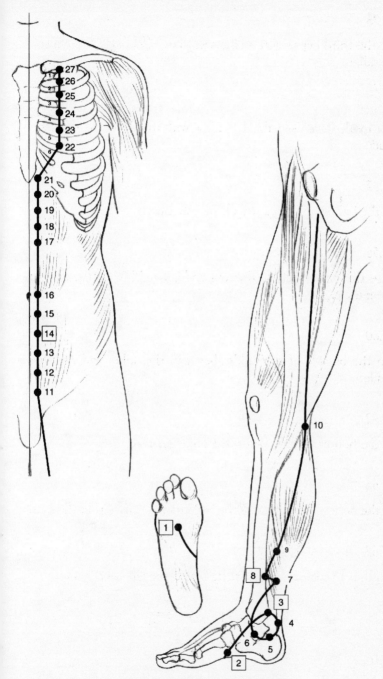

Figure 10   Kidney meridian (KD)

KD2

On the edge of the inside of the foot, in the arch.

KD3

Between the edge of the anklebone and the Achilles tendon, on the inside edge of the ankle.

KD6

Just below the anklebone.

KD14

To the side of and away two thumbs' width below the navel. The meridians on each side of the body are just one thumb's distance from each other.

Liver Meridian (LV)

LV1

Where the nail touches the flesh on the inside edge of the big toe.

LV2

On the front edge of the web between the big toe and second toe.

LV3

In the valley formed above the first and second toe.

LV8

On the inside of the knee, just above the crease formed when the knee is bent.

LV13

Just at the end of the floating eleventh rib.

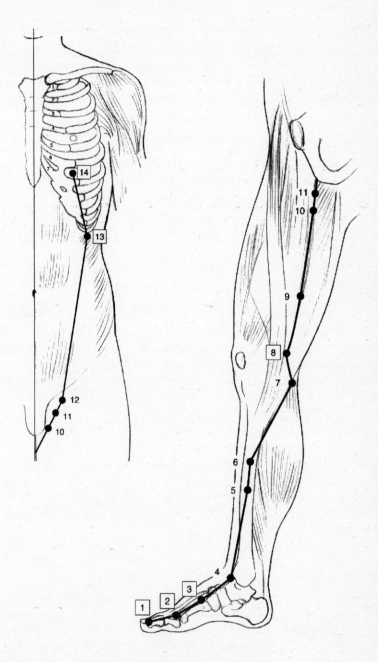

Figure 11   Liver meridian (LV)

LV14

Between the sixth and seventh ribs, directly below the nipple.

Gall Bladder Meridian (GB)

GB1

In the hollow at the edge of the eye socket.

GB8

Above the top of the ear, approximately one thumb's distance inside the hairline.

GB12

In the hollow at the base of the bone behind the ear.

GB18

Trace an arc with your thumb from the hairline to the base of the skull. Point found on the side of the head, above and behind the level of the ear, vertically above the neck muscles.

GB20

At the base of the skull, between the muscles.

GB21

In line with the seventh cervical vertebra, a little behind the highest point of the shoulder.

GB24

Directly below the nipple, in the cartilage between the seventh and eighth rib.

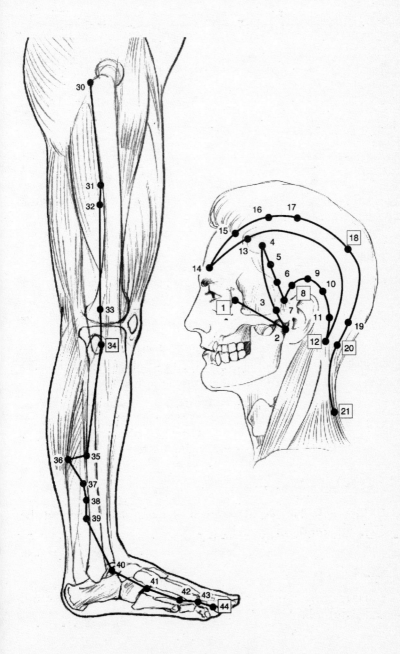

Figure 12 Gall bladder meridian (GB) (above and p 58)

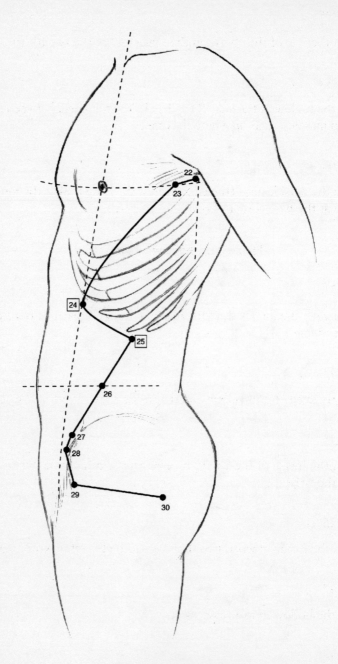

Gall bladder meridian (cont'd)

GB25

On the side of the chest, on the lower end of the twelfth rib.

GB34

In the hollow at the side of the leg, below the knee, between the two muscles, high up where they meet.

GB44

On the outside edge (the edge nearest the little toe) of the fourth toe at the base corner of the nail.

Heart Governor Meridian (HG)

HG1

Between the fourth and fifth ribs, one thumb's distance out from the nipple.

HG3

In the crease of the elbow, on the inside central part of the arm.

HG5

On the inside of the wrist, three fingers' width above the crease in the wrist.

HG6

On the inside of wrist, two thumb's width above the wrist crease.

HG7

In the hollow in the wrist joint.

HG8

In the centre of the palm.

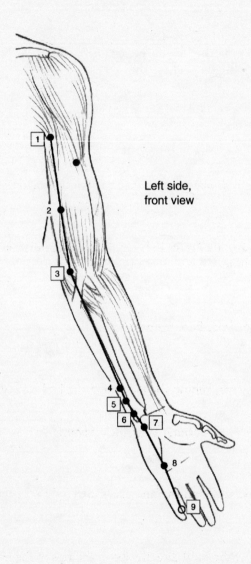

Left side,
front view

Figure 13   Heart governor meridian (HG)

HG9

On the middle finger at the base of the nail on the side nearest to the forefinger.

Triple Heater Meridian (TH)

TH1

On the outside edge of the fourth (ring) finger where the nail touches the flesh at the base.

TH4

In the hollow in the crease at the back of the hand.

TH5

On the back of the wrist, in the hollow between the bones of the radius and ulna.

TH17

At the base of the bone behind the ear.

TH20

Close to the ear, behind the ear and at the highest point.

Governing Vessel Meridian (GV)

GV16

Between the skull and the first cervical vertebra.

GV20

At the top of the skull directly above the tips of the ears.

GV24

On the middle of the head, just inside the hairline.

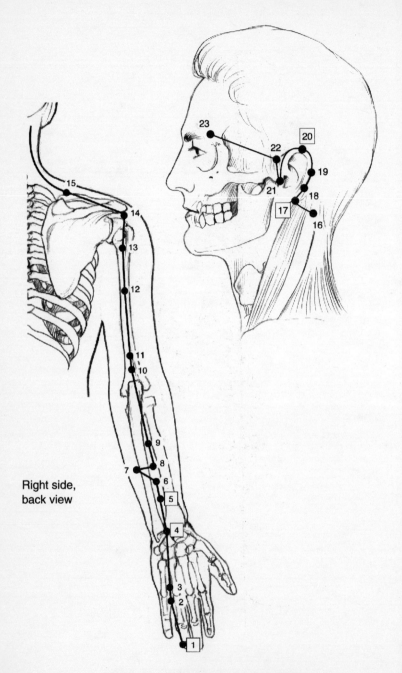

Right side,
back view

Figure 14 Triple heater meridian (TH)

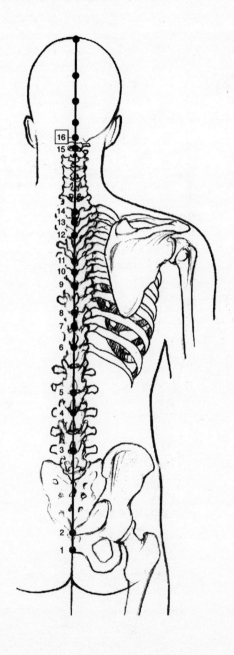

Figure 15 Governing vessel meridian (GV) (above and p 64)

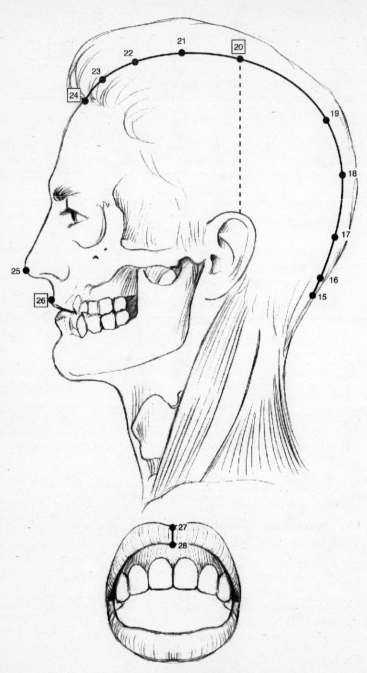

Governing vessel meridian

GV26

Below the nose, two-thirds of the way above the upper lip.

Conception Vessel Meridian (CV)

CV4

On the midline of the abdomen, four fingers' width below the navel.

CV6

On the midline of the abdomen, two fingers' width below the navel.

CV7

On the midline of the abdomen, one thumbs' width below the navel.

CV8

In the centre of the navel.

CV10

On the midline of the abdomen, two thumbs' width above the navel.

CV12

On the midline of the abdomen, four fingers' and one thumb's width above the navel.

CV14

On the midline of the abdomen, twice four fingers' width above the navel.

CV17

On the midline of the sternum, level with the nipples.

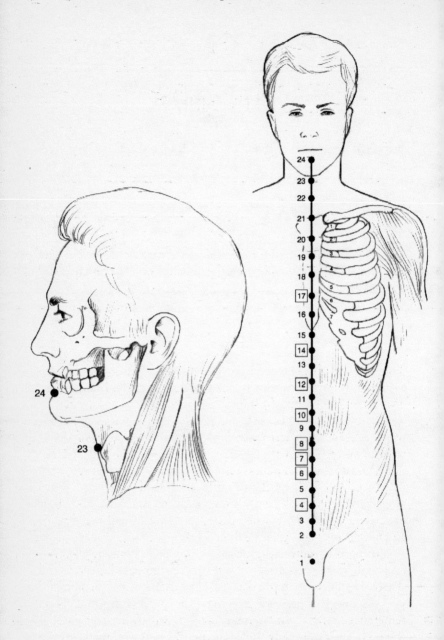

Figure 16   Conception vessel meridian (CV)

5

DIY Routines

THIS CHAPTER GIVES different routines for use in daily life. The first is based on the Japanese version of acupressure mentioned in the Preface.

DŌ-IN

The word *dō* in Japanese is the same as the Chinese word *tao* meaning 'the way'. *In* means being 'at home' or 'with ourselves'. This traditional form of Japanese self-massage was and is used by Zen Buddhist monks as they rise before dawn, samurai (Japanese warriors), shiatsu practitioners and martial artists. Its purpose is to bring us into line with our daily activity, like the activities we undertake in the early hours of the day to refresh us and invigorate us to face the day's challenge. When I travelled through Third World countries in the early 1970s, I always noticed a great buzz of activity around dawn when people were washing themselves or cleaning their space prior to their work.

During this routine, I would advise you to be more vigorous and apply more pressure if you want to be stimulated. Toward the end of the day or when you need to relax, then I would recommend you ease up the pressure and slow the process down. Always remember that the yin energy is rising up the front, soft parts of the body and conversely the yang energy is descending down the back and the harder parts of the body.

It is best to wear loose, comfortable cotton clothing, to be without your shoes and to have an empty stomach. You can begin either standing or sitting. If you stand, have your knees slightly bent and your feet parallel and about hip-width apart. If you sit in a chair have your feet firmly on the floor. You can also adopt the Japanese 'seiza' posture, which involves sitting on your knees with your buttocks resting on your heels and your toes touching. Choose whichever posture feels most comfortable and make sure you are not distracted. Let us begin!

- The tools for your practice of this acupressure workout are your hands. With relaxed shoulders, begin by placing your palms together at forehead height. Press your palms together and then begin to rub them vigorously and vertically (figure 17). Intersperse this activity with clapping once or twice abruptly. This process charges the chi in your hands and the clapping disperses all excess energy. After 30 seconds of rubbing shake out your hands, throwing away the energy towards the ground, shaking your wrists at the same time, and exhale sharply. Repeat this rubbing and shaking three or four times until your hands feel warm and tingly. Your chi energy is now flowing and you are ready for the routine.

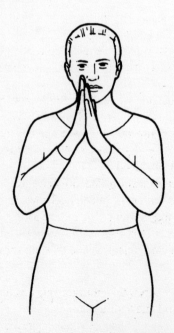

Figure 17   Rubbing the palms together

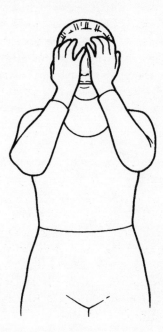

Figure 18 'Raking' the forehead

- With open hands and loose wrists begin by tapping all over your scalp as if you were drumming. Work on the top side and back of the head.
- Bring your fingertips to your forehead and rub vigorously up and down as if your fingers were a rake, from your hairline to your eyebrows (figure 18). Begin at the centre of your forehead and work towards your temples. (This stimulates the digestive system and gall bladder.)
- With your thumb and middle finger, pinch and squeeze your eyebrows from the centre of the eyebrows to the outside of the eyebrows. Try and achieve this in one long out-breath. Repeat this three times. (This area represents our lymphatic system – which is a slow and sluggish system that appreciates this kind of stimulation.)

These next three exercises stimulate our circulatory system, the lungs, the heart and the kidneys.

- Place your hands on your cheeks with the fingertips facing upwards. Press into the cheeks and at the same time rub up and down as fast as you can (figure 19). This exercise brings chi to the lung region.

- With the same vertical action rub either side of your nose. Repeat this for three out-breaths remembering that the more vigorous you are the more activating you are of the chi, in this case the heart chi.
- With the outside edge of your hands flick your ears from the back to the front. This is an energizing technique that stimulates the energy of the kidneys.
- With your thumb and middle finger press and squeeze BL1, which is found where the bridge of the nose meets the inside corners of the eyes (figure 20). Apply pressure as you breathe out and repeat this five more times. These points are very good for headaches behind the eyes and tired eyes.
- With your thumbs, work your way from the corner of the eyes along the upper eye socket until you find two small hollows that neatly fit your thumbs. Put the fleshy part of the thumb pad into the hollow, breathe in, and as you breathe out let the weight of your head drop forward on to your thumbs while

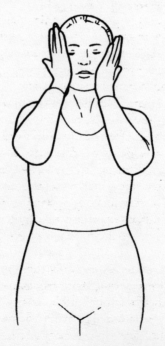

Figure 19 Pressing and rubbing the cheeks

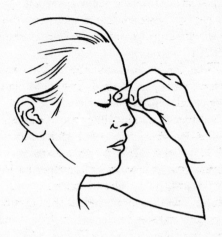

Figure 20   Squeezing BL1

resting your elbows on your chest to support the thumbs. This exercise stimulates BL2, which is useful for relieving headaches in the forehead region and sinus congestion.

- With your first and second fingers press into the eye socket on the lower portion (figure 21). Begin close to the eyes and work your way round to the far side, pressing five or six times. You can achieve this in one long out-breath. Repeat three times.

- Rotate your eyes as wide as possible in a clockwise direction, four or five times. Repeat this exercise in the opposite direction four or five times. Open your eyes as wide as possible so that there is a maximum stretch (yin). Screw up your face and eyelids (yang). These exercises strengthen the muscles of the eyes which relate to the function of the liver in oriental medicine.

- Now take hold of your ears, rotating them forwards, rotating them backwards, then pulling them forwards and pulling them backwards. Take hold of your earlobe and as you breathe out let the weight of your arm pull down. Hold on to the earlobes, breathe in and relax, then breathe out and let the weight pull down once more. Repeat this five or six times. This exercise strengthens our kidney energy and grounds us. This is a useful exercise if you feel tired during the day or distracted by too many things going on.

- Rotate your jaw as far as possible in one direction several times; repeat this in the opposite direction. Now try moving your jaw forwards then backwards. Chatter your teeth together and see if you can focus the pressure initially on the left side, then the centre, then the right side of the jaw. The mouth is the gateway to the digestive system and this helps strengthen the muscles in our mouth for chewing. It also activates our salivary glands that provide enzymes vital for the process of digestion.

- With your thumb and forefinger, pinch and squeeze the upper part of your lip. As you breathe out pull down towards the right side. Relax, breathe out and pull down towards the left side. The upper lip relates to the upper part of digestion – our stomach.

- Pinch and squeeze the central part of the lower lip, pulling the lower lip initially to the right then relax. Now pull the lower lip toward the left. Repeat this exercise three or four times. The

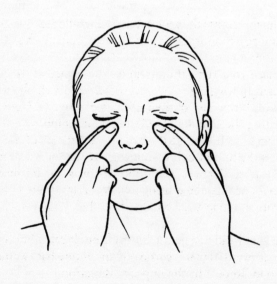

Figure 21 Pressing into the eye socket under the eyes

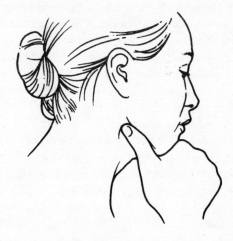

Figure 22   Working around the underneath of the jawbone

lower lip represents the function of the small intestine and large intestine again. This exercise will help circulate the blood and chi in that region.

- Now place your right thumb under the centre of the jawbone and begin to wiggle and press your way under the bone all the way towards the base of the right ear (figure 22). Here you are stimulating the salivary glands and your lymph nodes. Repeat this process with the left thumb on the left side of the jaw.
- Notice if the hollow below your ear is tender or not. If it is, this is often an indication of hardness or wax in the middle ear which can be alleviated using a little warm, filtered olive oil.
- Now rub and clap your hands, then shake out your hands as before.
- Rotate your head in a gentle but wide circle allowing your head to drop forward as you breathe out and rotate backwards as you breathe in. Repeat in the opposite direction.
- Link your fingers behind your head, raise your elbows and as you breathe out allow the weight of your hands and arms to pull your head down so that your chin touches your chest. Hold this

posture until you have completed your out-breath. Breathe in, raise your head and release the pressure. Repeat the exercise as you breathe out.

- With one hand on top of the other placed behind the neck, apply pressure at the base of the skull using the heel of your hand. Work your way down the neck towards the shoulder. This can alleviate pressure in the bladder and gall bladder meridians at the back and side of the neck.
- Stretch your right arm out so that your palm is facing forwards and your hand pointing towards the floor. With your left hand make a fist and, with a loose wrist, pound from the shoulder along the inside, softer part of the arm toward your open palm and the fingers of your right hand (figure 23). Work your way along the inside edge, the centre and outside edge of this softer, portion of the arm. Repeat this exercise three times. This exercise follows the heart, heart governor and lung meridians.
- Turn your hand over and keep your arm outstretched. Now pound from the back of the hand toward the shoulder, along the inside edge, the outside edge and along the centre of the

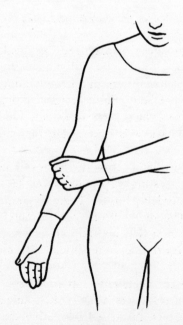

Figure 23   Pounding the inside of the arm

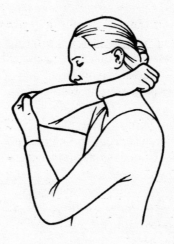

Figure 24   Pounding the shoulder

arm. This stimulates the small intestine, triple heater meridian and colon.

- Now rotate your right arm in a large windmill motion toward the front of your body. Build up more momentum and allow your breath to exhale the excess chi. Shake out your arm vigorously from the wrist and repeat this whole sequence with the left arm.

- Bring your right hand across the front of your body until your clenched fist is resting on your left shoulder, support your right elbow with your left palm and begin to pound gently into your left shoulder (figure 24). Work into the muscles and specifically focus on any area that appears tense or painful. Repeat this process now on the opposite shoulder. Remember to breathe out.

- With your back erect, tense up your fists, your wrists, your forearms, your shoulders, your neck, your jaw and your face. Make sure you have taken a deep breath in and hold the tension in this position for as long as you can. When you are ready, let go of the tension and the breath in one short exhalation. Repeat this exercise three times. The more temporarily we make ourselves yang (tight) the more it will help us relax and become yin as a result.

- Standing up, the backs of your legs straight, bend forward and bring your fists behind your back as far up as you can reach. Ideally, try and place the backs of your hands at the level of your shoulderblades. As you breathe out pound down either side of your spine toward the sacrum and then begin again as high up as you can reach (figure 25). Pound down and repeat this process at least four times. You are now working down the bladder meridian and you must avoid pounding directly on to the spine. Our bladder meridian and nervous system are vital for receiving chi energy and transmitting chi around the body. Any stretches or pressure we can apply to these areas help to keep us alert, focused and open to what lies ahead.

- Place the back of your right hand against the coccyx and your left hand with its palm facing down on top of your head. Simultaneously pound both up and down with pressure from both hands (figure 26). What this does in effect is to compress the chi energy through the centre of our body making us more alert. Do this process for one minute using the right hand and then switch hands for a further minute.

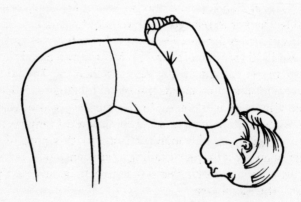

Figure 25 Pounding either side of the spine

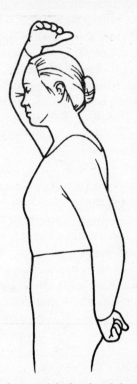

Figure 26 Pounding the top of the head and the coccyx simultaneously

- Make clenched fists, but maintain loose wrists and with the back of your hands pound the buttocks. Try and keep your shoulders and arms relaxed while you do this and find areas of sensitivity or tenderness. Deep into the hollows of each buttock is GB30 (*see* figure 12, p 57). Most of the blood that our system needs is used by the brain. When we lose focus or concentration it often means this blood is being used digesting a heavy meal or it is sitting in the muscles of the buttocks. This is an easy exercise to do even at work. Many years ago school teachers would apply pressure to this area of their pupils' anatomy if they were failing to concentrate! Conversely we can relax a person's nervous system by gently patting or rocking the sacral area.
- This next exercise is designed to stimulate and open up the lungs. The lung meridian begins just below the collarbone and works its way along the softer inside edge of the arm to the thumb (*see* figure 3, p 37). Begin by breathing in and

simultaneously stretching your arms with the palms facing forward so that your arms are now above your head at 45 degrees to your body. Hold the breath, look upwards and as you breathe out gently pound your chest in the region of LU1 and make a Tarzan call. Repeat this exercise four or five times or until your neighbours tell you to be quiet. The lungs play a vital part in the exchange of chi and we now live in a culture where they are not taxed to such a degree as they were in earlier times.

- Either sitting comfortably in your chair or kneeling in the seiza posture on the floor place your fingertips up under your ribs close to your sternum. As you breathe out lean forward and allow the back of your hand to rest on your thighs, thus driving your fingers gently up underneath the ribs (figure 27). This is not an exercise to do to someone else but is quite safe in your own hands. You will know how far to press. Breathe in and begin to sit up. Slide your fingers toward the central part of the ribs and again press up under the diaphragm and lean forwards. Finally place your fingertips on the outside edge of

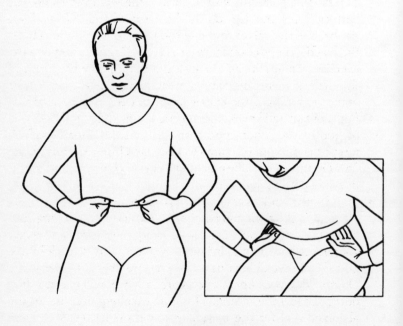

Figure 27 Pressing under the ribs

the ribs and repeat the process. This is an excellent massage for the internal organs (stomach, pancreas, spleen, liver and gall bladder).

- Sitting upright, place one hand upon the other with the underlying palm over the navel. With very little pressure gently rotate your hand in a clockwise direction around the navel. This calms and sedates the digestive system.

- Stand up for these next exercises. With your fists and wrists loose, pound down the outside of the legs from the hips to the outside of the ankle. This is the gall bladder meridian (*see* figure 12, p 57).

- Pound up the inside of the legs from the ankle along the centre of the calves, up the centre of the thighs toward the groin. This is the liver meridian (*see* figure 11, p 55). Pound down the front of the legs beyond the knees and on the outside edge of the shinbone toward the top of the foot. This is the stomach meridian (*see* figure 6, p 42–3). Now pound up the inside of the leg close to the shinbone, above the knee and up towards the groin. This is the spleen/pancreas meridian (*see* figure 5, p 41). Finally, pound down the back of the legs from where the buttock joins the leg, down the back of the knees, down the back of the calves to the outside edge of the ankle. This is the bladder meridian (*see* figure 9, p 50–1). Now complete the exercise by pounding up the inside of the leg from the inside of the ankle along the inside edge of the calf toward the inside edge of the groin. This is the kidney meridian (*see* figure 10, p 53).

- Put your feet and knees close together and cross your hands one on top of the other upon your knees. Bend your legs, look forward and rotate your ankles, knees and hips together (figure 28). Do this as low down as your knees will let you and repeat in the opposite direction.

- Stand with your legs as far apart as possible with your feet firmly planted on the floor and parallel to one another. Keeping your back straight and looking ahead bend your knees and lower your upper body to a point where you feel a stretch. Hold this posture for several breaths and then gently begin to rise again. Do not lock your knees and gently allow your knees to drop down and feel the stretch. This is an excellent exercise for the abdomen and for the meridians found on inside of the legs (liver, kidney, spleen/pancreas).

- While you are still standing, lift your right leg off the ground and shake it all about. Kick it forward, do a side kick and a mule kick behind you. Repeat this a few more times and then do the same exercise for the left leg and foot. This exercise helps eliminate stagnant chi from your body which may have built up during your exercise so far.

- Rub your hands and clap as in the opening routine and shake them out.
- Sit comfortably in a chair or on the floor and bring your right foot up so that your ankle is resting on your knee. Begin by rotating the ankle with your hand in large circles, clockwise then anticlockwise. With the back of your right hand pound from your big toe down towards the heel and along the soft, inside edge of the heel. Repeat this three times. Now rotate with your hands all the toes in turn clockwise and anticlockwise. At the end of the rotation take each toe in turn and squeeze and pull it on the out-breath to eliminate excess chi that has built up in the meridians. It is best to squeeze and pull upon the edges of the toe – this means where the nail joins the flesh on the edge (figure 29). This is more effective than holding

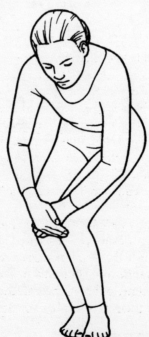

Figure 28   Rotating ankles, knees and hips together

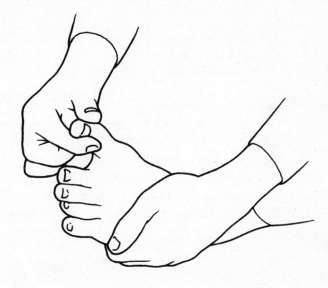

Figure 29   Squeezing the edges of the toes

the toe above and below. Complete this exercise with the foot by slapping the foot hard on to the floor.

- Stretch both legs out in front of you. Notice the difference between them. The right leg that you have massaged will feel vibrant, alive and tingly whereas your left leg which you have yet to work on will feel cold, lifeless and lacking in energy. This is a great moment to reflect how we are generally when we have not done any dō-in. We often wander around like our left leg.
- To complete the sequence, massage your left ankle, sole and toes.
- Rub and shake out your hands vigorously again.
- Sit comfortably with your eyes closed and allow your breathing to come from your belly. You could place your hands over the navel to help you tune into your breath. Feel yourself sink into the floor. Have a sense of being there in the moment and then begin to visualize the activities that you are about to pursue.

Yang Visualization

If the activities ahead of you involve you being clear and focused and active then I would suggest that at the end of your DIY acupressure routine you try this kind of visualization.

With your eyes closed, imagine that rotating in front of you about 1 yard (metre) away is a large uncut diamond. Spend a few minutes admiring its qualities. Absorb its qualities and, if you like, be its qualities. As we perceive the nature of this diamond we can begin to take on its characteristics when we return to our day-to-day activity. For example we can be clear, focused, incisive, reliable and durable. Slowly begin to open your eyes and notice the effect on your energy.

Yin Visualization

If the activities ahead of you involve you being more relaxed, open and creative then try this visualization.

With your eyes closed take yourself to a special place that you have visited at some point in your life. It is not unusual that this place is in nature and has charming peaceful qualities that you felt inspired by at the time and that you have never forgotten. Try and imagine yourself in that space and absorb the qualities of the environment that so inspired you at the time. Let that environment envelope your chi. You remain in this restful, peaceful state as you slowly open your eyes.

It is only by practising regularly this form of DIY acupressure that you begin to feel its benefits. You could take a few minutes in the morning or evening or even during your break to try it. It is a wonderful way to be in touch with your body and I hope that you can share it with your family and friends.

ACUPRESSURE FOR SPECIFIC MERIDIANS

What follows is a specific outline for working on each of the meridians. Use appendix 2 to find out the meridian or meridians to which you need to give attention. What is worth noting is that you must work on both sides of the body and that it is wise to massage and give acupressure to the associated partner meridian (see table 3, p 32). For example, if you feel that you have many symptoms associated with a liver imbalance do not forget to pay just as much attention to the meridian of the gall bladder. These meridians work in harmony and it is inevitable that if there is a problem in one you will feel discomfort in the other.

You will notice from the acu point diagrams in chapter 4 that many of the points are towards the periphery of the body. This is because when we developed in embryo our limbs sprouted like buds from the trunk. As these limbs grew and developed they brought with them the charge and energy from the deepest part of the body from where they originated. Consequently there is a concentration of points around the hands, fingers and wrists as well as the toes, feet and ankles. If you look carefully at your arms and legs you will notice that they have a more spiral-like structure with a more focused and concentrated development at the periphery. By working on the hands and feet in particular you are awakening the chi in the organs on a deep level.

What now follows is a simple routine for each of the meridians. If you find it difficult to locate the points described see the diagrams in chapter 4.

Lung Meridian

Stretch your left arm out to your side with your palm facing forwards and bring the middle finger of your right hand to the clavicle. Feel down below the clavicle until you meet the first rib and find the gap between the first and second rib. The point (LU1) is usually tender. Breathe out and apply pressure. Bend your elbow and make a fist until the tendon on the elbow is taut. Find the hollow on the outside/thumb side of the elbow close to the tendon and apply pressure into this hollow (LU5). Come to the point where the wrist meets the hand, flex your hand forward and back and with the thumb of your right hand find the hollow at the base of the hand (LU9). Where the bottom of the thumbnail touches the flesh of the thumb on the softer part of the hand apply pressure with your right thumb or right thumbnail (LU11).

Large Intestine Meridian

Pinch and squeeze the outside edge of the forefinger where the nail touches the flesh (LI1). Come up the valley in between the forefinger and the thumb, find the fleshy mound, and as you breathe out apply pressure at the head of the valley between the forefinger and the thumb (LI4). Bend your elbow so that your arm is lying across the front of your body at 90 degrees to the upper arm. Notice where the crease appears on the elbow. Trace along until the end of this crease and then go immediately down to the bone below. Press hard against the bone on the upper section of the bone LI11. Using your forefinger press into the depression next to the nose where it joins the cheek (LI20).

Spleen/Pancreas Meridian

When observing the spleen/pancreas meridian, make sure there is no hard skin on the inside edge of the big toe. This prevents chi from rising along the meridian and should be removed by whatever method is recommended to you by an expert. Begin by measuring using three of your own fingers' width above the anklebone, bring the thumb of your opposite hand across and apply pressure close to the bone (S/P6). Next, keeping your thumb in position shift your three fingers above your thumb, resting them against the bone, and bring the thumb of your left hand above these three fingers (S/P7). Keeping your left thumb in place, measure again above using the three fingers of your other hand, move your thumb above and this is S/P8. Keeping your thumb in place measure now a further three fingers which will bring you into the hollow below the knee (S/P9). Finally, move above the knee on to the muscle above the knee but on the inside part of the leg. S/P10 is close to the bone and can be extremely painful.

Stomach Meridian

Bring the palm of your right hand across so that it is facing down on to your left kneecap. Where the middle finger of your right hand touches the outside edge of the shinbone you will find ST36. Bring your left thumb across and apply pressure to this area. Bend and flex your foot and locate the hollow were the foot joins the leg (ST41). Find the highest point of bone on the upper foot (ST42). Finally massage and squeeze and pull the second and third toe (ST45).

Heart Meridian

With your left arm relaxed at your side and your palm facing forwards, bring your right thumb across and press deep into the front part of the armpit (HT1). Bend the elbow and on the outside edge of the soft part of the elbow locate HT3. Bend and flex the wrist and in the hollow where the hand joins the arm find HT7. Finally, where the nail touches the flesh on the inside edge of the small finger apply pressure using either the thumb or the nail of your right hand (HT9).

Small Intestine Meridian

With your arm relaxed by your side and with the back of your hand facing forward squeeze and press the small fingertip particularly where the nail touches the flesh on the outside edge (SI1). Bend and flex the wrist and in the hollow between the arm and the hand find SI5. Flex your elbow and discover the hollow on the outside edge of the elbow where SI8 is located.

Bladder Meridian

With your left leg relaxed and the muscles loose at the back of the leg, place one thumb on top of the other and trace your way down the back of the calf until you discover BL57. You can flex the muscles to discover the hollow where it can be found. On the outside edge of the ankle behind the anklebone and next to the Achilles tendon you can discover BL60. Pinch and squeeze this between your thumb and forefinger. (*Do not use this point during pregnancy.*) Pinch and squeeze the end of the small toe (BL67). (*Do not use this point during pregnancy.*)

Kidney Meridian

With the sole of your foot upturned towards you, apply pressure in the valley between the hard skin below the big toe and the remaining four toes (KD1). Trace your way along the softer part of the foot until you find KD2 which is located midway along the arch of the foot. Using the outside edge of both of your hands rub vigorously on the inside and outside of your ankle which helps to stimulate the energy of KD3, 4, 5 and 6.

Liver Meridian

Massage the inside edge of the big toe, particularly where the nail joins the flesh (LV1). Work your way up the valley between the big toe and the second toe and massage LV2. Move up the calf now to behind the knee on the inside edge of the large tendon (LV8).

Gall Bladder Meridian

Bring your right thumb over to the outside of your left leg. Locate GB34 in the hollow where the two muscles join below the knee on the outside of the leg. A good way to find this point is to flex the muscles and apply pressure on the out-breath. Complete by massaging the fourth toe (GB44). Squeeze and pull as you breathe out.

Heart Governor Meridian

With the palm of your hand facing forwards and your arm relaxed by your side, find your way down the edge of the ribcage below the collarbone until you meet the fifth rib. Press this with your middle finger (HG1). Bend your elbow, flex the muscles of your left palm and bring your right thumb across the inside edge of the tendon that appears and press into the hollow (HG3). Three fingers' width above the crease on the inside edge of the wrist at the centre of the wrist, find HG5. Where the hand joins the forearm, in the middle of the crease, find HG7. At the centre of the palm press deeply (HG8). Locate the point on the middle finger of your left hand where the nail touches the flesh on the side of the middle finger closest to the forefinger. Press hard with the thumb of your right hand or the thumbnail of your right hand (HG9).

Triple Heater Meridian

Massage the tip of the ring finger of your left hand, particularly the edge closest to the small finger (TH1). Let your arm hang by your side with the back of the hand facing forward, flex the wrist, and where the hand joins the arm, midway across the join press TH4. Three fingers' width above the crease between the two bones of the wrist on the back of the arm press TH5.

Governing Vessel Meridian

Gently rock your head forward and back then bring the forefinger of your right hand to the point were the skull joins the neck (GV16). Bring the middle finger of your right hand to the very top of your head and press (GV20). Place the palm of your hand against the side of your head above your ear as support. Rest your palms on your forehead and press deeply on the hairline (GV24). With the thumb of your right hand, find the point two-thirds of the distance up between your upper lip and the base of your nose (GV26).

Conception Vessel Meridian

Measure three fingers' width below your navel with your left hand, bring the middle finger of your right hand across and press in as you breathe out (CV6). Measure two fingers' width directly down from the tip of the sternum and press (CV14). Directly below the lower lip apply pressure against the gum (CV24).

6

Where to Go from Here

WHILE THE PRECEDING chapters give you an insight into the origins of acupressure and points for relief of aches and pains, it is wise to look at the underlying cause of a problem should it keep repeating and to take preventative action. Indeed many people who have benefited from acupressure for various ailments are encouraged to go deeper into the whole process. To study acupuncture or Chinese herbal medicine in detail is an awesome undertaking so this chapter summarizes their recommendations and insights and makes them appropriate to this day and age.

Chinese medicine was originally designed to be a preventative system and practitioners encourage their patients to keep themselves in harmony with nature through their diet, activity, breathing and adaptation to the changes in seasons and weather. The following extract from the *Nei Ching*, written by the Yellow Emperor in approximately 2600 BC gives us an insight into this philosophy.

Those who rebel against the basic rules of the universe sever their own roots and ruin their true selves. Yin and yang, the two princi-ples in nature, and the four seasons are the beginning and the end of everything and they are also the cause of life and death. Those who disobey the laws of the universe will give rise to calamities and visitations, while those who follow the laws of the universe remain free from dangerous illness, for they are the ones who have obtained Tao, the Right Way.

Hence the sages did not treat those who were already ill; they instructed those who were not yet ill. They did not want to rule those who were already rebellious; they guided those who were not rebellious. To administer medicines to diseases which have already developed and to suppress revolts which have already developed is comparable to the behaviour of those persons who begin to dig a well after they have become thirsty. Would these actions not be too late?

The Yellow Emperor criticizes 'modern lifestyle', pointing out that:

> ... in ancient times the people lived in harmony, but nowadays [some five thousand years ago] people are not living according to the seasons, eating what is local and available, they are erratic in their behaviour and sleep and they spend more time amusing themselves and less time in self-reflection and prayer.

LOOKING AT OUR LIVES AS A WHOLE

What has fascinated me most in the past 20 years is how our health is reflected in many facets of our lives. Therefore, when symptoms reappear or become stubborn or manifest later, but in a slightly different form, it is wise to be curious as to why this pattern keeps repeating itself. A busy lifestyle can distract us from really listening to our body but it is probably even more important now than in the past to listen to ourselves on a regular basis. In some cultures this would have been called prayer or self-reflection. Today we perhaps call it meditation or visualization. Another way to get an honest answer about your current state is to ask the opinion of a friend who appears robust and grounded.

Take a plant, for example. If the leaves of a plant become dry and brittle then it is clear that most of the problem lies with the root structure and the soil nursing the plant, rather than external influences, like the air. The best way to remedy the problem is obviously to add more water to the soil or use different soil. Dealing with the problem purely externally, sponging or spraying the leaves, would bring a symptomatic result but would do little to prevent the situation from recurring.

I heard a wonderful definition of insanity which I believe puts in context the importance of dealing with the cause rather than the symptoms: insanity is to repeat a process but expect a different result – rather like putting your finger in a door frame, slamming the door and experiencing serious pain but believing that if you repeat the process it will not hurt. So many times we can make this fundamental mistake in our lives. Even the most intelligent amongst us. It appears to be a modern human characteristic to look for symptomatic relief from health problems, environmental problems, economic problems and emotional problems. It takes far more work, far more courage and far more commitment to dig down to the roots of the problem and begin deep, organic change.

Ten years ago a unique project was begun at a leading London hospital involving men who had experienced their first heart attack. As they recovered in hospital the men were given two choices of treatment. The first choice involved the use of medication and a period of observation in hospital after which they were free to return home and go back to work. They could probably achieve this in 10 to 20 days. No change was required to their lifestyle or to their diet. They were also told that they would probably have another heart attack and that it would most likely be fatal. The second option offered to the men was the opportunity to remain longer in the hospital and reinvent themselves on many different levels. They would be coached in how to relax by using meditation and visualization. They would face fundamental questions about the level of stress in their lives and how to change this in a radical way once they had returned to their work or home. They were also encouraged to learn how to relax by singing and dancing and spontaneous artistic expression. They were then told that their diet needed reviewing and a reduction in saturated animal fat and sugar would be beneficial. This whole process would detain them longer, perhaps for weeks, but on returning home they were assured it would be unlikely they would have another heart attack. The choice was theirs. Which did most of them favour? It seems unbelievable but most men favoured the first choice.

We begin now by looking at some of the factors that we have control over in our daily lives and that can be related to the symptoms, aches and pains from which we are seeking relief. Remember that as you read, it is important to see yourself in the biggest possible perspective. What I mean is, if you constantly have yang-type symptoms then look for the areas of excessive yang in your life. Similarly this argument holds true of chronic yin symptoms – you would need to look at what can bring more yang into your life.

Diet

What we eat on a daily basis is probably the most important factor in determining our blood quality, energy levels and general well-being. In the era of the Yellow Emperor there were probably only about three hundred varieties of food available to the people. On the whole, they ate what was local and what was in season and adjusted the cooking style to suit the season. There is a lot to be said even in this day and age for keeping our diet relatively modest and adjusting it to fit with our climate. Now, some five thousand years later there are over 2,500 food additives alone for our bodies to assimilate.

What is important to remember is that you and I have a choice. One of the principles I encourage is to eat foods that have integrity. This means that whenever possible prepare foods that are organic and that have been processed in a minimal fashion. Even if your lifestyle does not give you much time for the preparation of natural and whole foods, it is still wise to take time when the seasons change to simplify your diet and allow any elimination of excess that has built up.

Food and the Seasons

Practically speaking during the fire season (summer) we need to eat more salads than usual, more fruit, more pulses – foods that are generally lighter and require less cooking. It is only common sense that if we eat roast and baked animal food with plenty of salt in combination with stews and soups which have been cooked for hours, we will be too hot, too heavy and too yang to feel comfortable during this season.

During the adjustment towards autumn (soil) it is wiser for us to begin to use a slower, settling form of cooking such as boiling and to increase the amount of time used in the cooking process itself. Appropriate foods include pumpkins and other squashes (eg marrows), grains (eg rice) and the sweeter and harder fruits that have become available at this time.

As we move into the deep autumn (metal) our bodies require more heat and more richness of food to help us draw in our chi to face the onset of winter.

During the water season (winter) in a four-season climate, we need to use long cooking methods and more salt to balance the excess of cold (yin) and the pernicious damp of winter. It is unwise to live on a diet dominated by raw fruit and salad at this time.

In the spring, or when the energy of wood is present, we can begin to make our diet more yin in order to help loosen the stagnation and grip of winter. This means making our cooking shorter with plenty of steaming and light sautéing. Beneficial also at this time of year is fasting and using sharp-tasting pickles to activate the liver and digestive system.

Food and Daily Activity

Other considerations around diet are to do with matching what you eat with your daily activity. There is no point eating more than you need. In fact it is excess food which causes much disease. A breakfast of bacon and eggs may well be burnt off by an individual who is physically active all morning in the construction industry. Although the food is high in saturated fat and salt the activities that they are pursuing uses up the food. Conversely, having this kind of breakfast and then being engaged for the day in an intellectual pursuit with no physical activity at all leads to stagnation. The secret is to design and enjoy food that fits our purpose in life, our current condition and our basic constitution.

Recreation

Designing and engaging in an activity which balances our usual mode of living is the real purpose of recreation. When you look at the word it actually means re-creation, suggesting that the activity should inspire and recharge us. In an ideal world, we choose the kinds of activities that give us the polarity we need. However, often we are attracted to the very activity that increases the imbalance within us. It is not unusual for example if we have a more yang nature and more yang activity in our jobs that we will be most comfortable practising sports that endorse this, like squash, badminton, rugby, soccer and other team sports. What we often need when we are too yang is really the opposite but it does not fit into our frame of thinking. The thought of meditation, tai chi, yoga or aromatherapy when we are in yang mode is probably impossible. If on the other hand we are tired, unenthusiastic, distracted and apathetic, we may not be attracted to the yang activity we need and prefer to find a pursuit that requires little physical effort and minimal social interaction. However, it is only by stretching ourselves physically and emotionally that we can regain some balance.

Physical Exercise

I do not believe there are any rules about recreation or physical activity, but it is important to remember that less than one hundred years ago we had no cars or central heating and people kept more physically active as a result. Some strong physical activity that gets us breathless and sweaty at least three times a week is advisable. If a level of excitement or thrill can be built into the programme, so much the better. This helps both to stimulate and to discharge the energy and tension present in the body. Think back to the last time you were very excited about something and to how elated and refreshed you felt later.

Rather than make your recreational activity more of the same, try to design an activity that helps you balance your lifestyle. Initially, it can take some effort, but use your intuition in designing what will work – perhaps by drawing up a list of all the activities that are possible or that you have participated in during your life or that you have always promised yourself to try. Try a few of these so that you can build up a menu of different activities to choose from at different times as your needs vary.

Relaxation

The greatest demands on modern human beings are to the nervous system. In ancient times we needed a sharp nervous system for our hunting and gathering, but today this sensitivity is overtaxed. The constant ringing of the telephone, the noise of traffic, the information we receive via radio, television and newspapers all induce stress within the system. We have devised various ways of releasing this stress such as participating in or watching various sports or listening to music but sometimes this stress is released through violent or strange behaviour.

Recreation for the nervous system and mind can be achieved through different kinds of meditation. Some people find it difficult to sit quietly for 10 or 15 minutes simply concentrating on their breath and may prefer the more active versions of meditation such as tai chi or chi kung. I encourage you to discover what works for you by trying out the variety of meditation and visualization techniques that are available. Remember also what we call ourself. We call ourself a 'human being' and it is a return to this state of 'being' that can relax the nervous system completely. We seem to be moving away from the human being into more of a 'human doing'. Rediscovering this quality of being 'in the moment' is the essence of all meditation systems.

Feng Shui

Growing in popularity in the West is feng shui which is essentially understanding our home or office space as a reflection of ourselves. As with acupressure, feng shui is based on having a harmonious and free flowing distribution of chi throughout our space, with different areas of our houses relating to different aspects of our lives. In a similar way to acupressure we are looking for areas which have become blocked or stagnant and make adjustments to our space in order to allow this chi to flow unimpeded. With the use of crystals, plants, mirrors or light we can enhance areas of our home where the chi is stuck. Stagnation is often reflected in our health, our wealth, our relationships and our finances. It is therefore important to find the stagnation in all areas. As with acupressure, you will only receive symptomatic relief by making adjustments and it is more important to look at the big picture to see what is the cause of the problem and how to bring about those changes.

The use of acupressure in our lives could be called 'inner feng shui' since both systems emanate from the same philosophy and they can be successfully used hand in hand. If you have persistent and chronic difficulties with your health it is well worth investigating whether chi is moving well in your home or workplace. There are a number of books on the subject as well as many professional practitioners who can advise.

WHAT IS HEALTH?

This is a fascinating question to ask any student at a seminar on natural healing. The frequent response is that health is the absence of disease. What you rarely hear is a list of symptoms associated with good health. Years ago I came across a definition of health by George Ohsawa, a Japanese teacher and philosopher who went to Europe in the 1920s, and I find it an inspiring reminder of what to aim at. He lists seven levels of health, beginning with the easier ones to change and progressively getting more challenging. You will perhaps notice that many people have problems with the first two or three and that these are also the ones that begin to improve when we initiate changes in our health and lifestyle. Ohsawa's definition of the seven levels of health is as follows.

Never Tired

All of us can feel tired from time to time but chronic tiredness pervades all aspects of our lives.

Good Appetite

This is not just for food but for life itself. The individuals on our planet with the greatest appetite are children. They are constantly hungry and curious. It is really this curiosity that is one of the essential qualities of good health.

Good Memory

On one level this is the mechanical process that helps us to remember names and telephone numbers, but equally it can be the biological memory that we all have within us. It is the memory deep within ourselves of what it is to be healthy and the memory present within the organs of the body that allow them to fulfil their function efficiently. Ill-health and disease often occur because of a kind of cellular amnesia or because we are not in touch with what our bodies are recording.

Good Sleep

Good sleep is deep and restful and uninterrupted by nightmares or the need to visit the bathroom. There is no set amount of sleep required, only that it is sufficient and leaves us charged and enthusiastic for the new day.

A Sense of Humour

This is vital. Humour is our mental and physical flexibility which helps to make balance within the stresses and strains of modern living. When we succumb to the pressures and lose our vitality, flexibility and humour we are beginning to develop more serious problems.

Being Joyful and Alert

This level is concerned with the state of our nervous system. We can observe it in our eyes and in our expression, in much the same way as we diagnose the freshness of a fish in the marketplace. Dull eyes and a dull expression are indications of apathy and imbalance. Trust and joy are fundamental to good health.

Gratitude

Ohsawa said this was the single most important factor in our health. Gratitude in this context is accepting unconditional responsibility for our lives and the events we have created. The opposite to this way of thinking is the feeling of being a victim all the time. When we begin to accept responsibility for our health and for changing our health we can begin to be truly healthy.

I hope these ideas will leave you hungry for more and I encourage you to practise or try many of the ancillary systems that I have mentioned as well as acupressure. This will hopefully give you access to a far wider picture of oriental healing – which I believe has an enormous contribution to make to humanity at this time. I believe that collective responsibility for our environment, our future and our children begins by taking individual responsibility and that acupressure and its associated disciplines make an excellent starting place. I wish you good health and peace.

Appendix 1

Case Histories

ACUPRESSURE REALLY COMES into its own when we are called upon to use it in emergencies. I am grateful to my background in dō-in and aikido as these help to ground me quickly in first aid situations. It is at these times that you are really guided by intuition and not by a manual.

Do remember that if you encounter a problem where you feel that your acupressure could bring relief ask the person if they mind you treating them.

What follows now are a few situations where I found acupressure helpful. Perhaps you can relate to some of these experiences and will be able use these stories as useful starting points for yourself.

CHILDBIRTH

My first wife, Marion, and I were both shiatsu students and given that she was also a midwife we both opted for home births for our children. We had always heard in class how certain points were not to be used during pregnancy as they can cause miscarriage, for example SP6 and BL60, and we were keen to use acupressure in labour in order to avoid using pethidine or any other form of artificial pain control. My wife had tended many women during childbirth and she knew she wished to be fully alert during labour. As with many first labours hers went on for hours and hours and after some 20 hours with a very patient and understanding midwife at home it became clear that she was getting tired and the cervix was no longer dilating. The midwife said that the baby was not showing any signs of distress but if labour did not progress she would have to go to hospital and be induced.

At this stage my wife and I discussed together the option of using acupressure points to speed up the labour and the midwife agreed to give us half an hour. It was then that I began to massage S/P6 on both ankles and with increasing vigour. After several minutes I moved on to BL67 (at the point where the outside edge of the nail meets the flesh on the edge of the foot). Squeezing this part of the toe as hard as I could between my thumb and forefinger I then moved on to start using my thumbnail.

After some 15 minutes the midwife announced that things were on the move and that the birth was imminent. Marion had always wished to give birth squatting and this gives access to BL27, 28 and 29 on the sacrum. These points alleviate lower back pain and relax the pelvis and lower back. With your thumbs either side of the spine and held in the indentations along the sacrum you can get tremendous pressure on the person's out-breath. I found that it was relatively easy to apply the pressure as the contractions came. Our son was delivered quite successfully half an hour later and Marion was able to say that the bladder points on the sacrum really helped to diminish the pain.

If you were to interview a hundred women and ask them what their labours were like you would get a hundred very different responses. This case history is only meant as a guide to what we did and you may find aspects of it useful in your situation. What was really apparent to me was the importance of breathing and using the pressure on the person's out-breath.

PANIC ATTACK

This is a very distressing situation which many people experience during their lives. It is not necessarily brought on by acute fear or a dangerous situation, but can be connected with an inability to breathe properly. When you look at the physical symptoms of panic attack you will notice that they have a lot in common with those of hyperventilation. The symptoms of both a panic attack and hyperventilation include: fast heartbeat, heart palpitations, irregular heartbeat, dizziness, headaches, tension, blurred vision, anxiety, sighing, yawning, twitching in the muscles,

tiredness, sweating and a feeling of being outside your body.
We normally breathe in two different ways.

1 When we exercise strongly we use our chest muscles, and these
   stretch the ribs allowing us a larger capacity of air into the lungs
   than normal.
2 In relaxed and restful situations we tend to use our diaphragm
   which is the sheet of muscle which divides the chest from the
   abdominal cavity. Usually this raises and lowers itself putting
   pressure on to the lungs to help breathe out.

It is not uncommon to find that in a panic attack the diaphragm
has gone into a form of spasm. One of my shiatsu students would
regularly experience panic attacks while travelling on the underground railway to class and one morning appeared late for the
session clearly in great distress. She was frightened, breathless,
sweaty and at a loss to know what to do. I got her to lie comfortably
on her back and began to work on HG6 (which is to be found one
thumb's width above the wrist crease on the central, inside part
of the arm). This point on both wrists is perfect to begin to calm
anyone in a stressful situation. I then began to work on ST41
(which is located on the stomach meridian on the outside of the
shinbone and in the hollow where the bone meets the foot – you
can find this on yourself by raising and lowering your foot until
you find the hollow which neatly fits your thumb). This is an
excellent point for taking the spasm out of the diaphragm.

I worked on both feet for some five minutes and I was later able
to show her what to do for future situations. Since she also had
these attacks frequently and could bring them on herself by
thinking 'I am about to have another panic attack', I suggested
that she saw a therapist who could help her trace the pattern in
her memory that was the deep-seated cause of the problem. What
also helps in such situations is a re-education of the breathing
using yoga or tai chi.

FAINTING

As in most first aid situations, if someone fainted I would begin
with HG6 and then move on to GV26. This is a point which is
found between the upper portion of the upper lip and where the
nose joins the face above it. Midway between the two ridges that

run vertically you will find the point two-thirds of the way up in the groove. It is easier to press this point with your forefinger and a mild effect can by achieved by rubbing horizontally with the outside edge of your forefinger. I tried these successfully on a lady who fainted shortly after getting off a bus in London that I was about to board. Having asked if there was a nurse or doctor around I then went on to begin massaging HG6 which to most onlookers appeared as if I was checking her pulse. What really brought her round was the pressure on GV26 and if you try pressing this on yourself you will see why it rouses most people.

It was pointed out to me by a Japanese teacher that our nervous systems have developed from the early vertebrates – fish – and that the most powerful part of the fish's nervous system is the very front. This is its sensor. The very tip of their nose appears in our structure at GV26. If you ever need to dispatch a fish very quickly and efficiently, you hit it very hard in this region. Similarly, if you are hit extremely hard just below the nose it can knock you out and conversely if you are stimulated hard (hit in this area, but not very hard) it can instantly wake you up and make you more alert. That is also why being slapped in the face can instantly make you very alert. So be careful in a fist fight that you don't make your opponent more aggressive by stimulating them in GV26!

TRAVEL SICKNESS

This can affect anyone and even Lord Nelson was known to suffer with seasickness! I suggest that initially you use HG6 – the wrist bands on sale in recent years for travel sickness perpetually stimulate this point. I then recommend working on ST36. Remember that this point also helps give us renewed energy, useful in travel sickness as one of its side effects is lethargy and sleepiness.

The other point that I have found useful with travel sickness is LV2 (which can be found one thumb's width up from the crease between the big toe and the second toe). It is neatly positioned in the valley between the two bones and you can press this fairly hard on the out-breath. This helps ground a person's energy and since nausea is a yin manifestation it helps to stabilize and yangize their condition.

From a martial arts point of view, travel sickness is associated with a temporary weakness in the 'hara'. The hara is regarded in

Japan as our centre and is located two fingers' width below the navel. If you spread-eagle yourself you will notice that you pivot on the hara. By bringing our breathing into this region and keeping it warm we can help strengthen it.

A traditional Japanese remedy for travel sickness is to fill the navel with salt and strap it in place with a plaster, as this yanizes the area. While travelling to and from a conference in Holland by sea with students several years ago, one of them had a very bad crossing. Before returning he was determined to avoid seasickness. He tried the advice and was the life and soul of the party despite the rough seas. He looked so dishevelled when we landed in the UK that Customs picked him out for a more in depth discussion. A closer search of him revealed the salt which was sent for tests and he was delayed for two hours.

Appendix 2

Quick Reference to Oriental Diagnosis

T HIS IS JUST INTENDED as a taste of what is possible with diagnosis and I encourage you to watch and observe colleagues, friends and family as well as seeing debates and current affairs programmes on the television with a new eye. What follows should help you pinpoint areas of weakness that you can work on with the help of chapters 4 and 5. It details each meridian, its physiology and function, what damages or supports the related systems and some of the indications of imbalance. With this background information on physiology from an oriental perspective and a fundamental understanding of yin and yang it will be possible for you to approach symptoms you may have.

Liver (Yang Organ) (Yin Meridian)

Physiology Seen as a compact and active organ. Stores and provides energy for our muscles. An elimination organ.
Damaged by Late-night eating; alcohol; eating too quickly or when distracted; stress; oversleeping in the morning.
Supported by Physical activity, pickles, stretching, dancing, laughter.
Diagnosis Irritability, anger, stiffness in the joints especially elbows and knees.

Gall Bladder (Yin Organ) (Yang Meridian)

Physiology A hollow inactive organ supplying bile to the digestive tract. Mainly used to emulsify fats and oils.
Damaged by Excessive amounts of fat and oil; large amounts of spice; very cold liquids and cold dairy products; draughts; planning and thinking ahead all the time; stress.
Supported by Pickles, good-quality vinegar.
Diagnosis Constantly planning, hypersensitive to draughts, noises and strong smells.

Heart (Yang Organ) (Yin Meridian)

Physiology Seen as the centre of our circulatory system and as governing the rhythm of our lives.
Damaged by Excessive amounts of salt and animal foods; chaotic or erratic lifestyle; no rhythm in our lives.
Supported by Having rhythm in our lives. Good-quality exercise and laughter.
Diagnosis Erratic behaviour. Poor circulation in the hands and feet. Sometimes a ruddy complexion or a swollen nose.

Small Intestine (Yin Organ) (Yang Meridian)

Physiology This is where we absorb our nutrients. Involved in the process of elimination.
Damaged by Excessive amounts of salt and hard indigestible baked flour products (eg biscuits and dry crackers); tension – getting 'knotted up'.
Supported by Chewing very well. Modest amounts of sea vegetables in the diet. Exercise that tones the abdomen.
Diagnosis Deep vertical lines on the side of the head close to the ear.

Spleen/Pancreas (Yang Organ) (Yin Meridian)

Physiology These organs are seen as partners in Chinese medicine. They are connected with storage of energy and form the foundation of our immune system.

Damaged by Dairy food and sugar; being constantly criticized; feeling anxious, insecure and worried about the future.
Supported by Good-quality sweet-tasting foods including fruits, root vegetables and round vegetables. Grain malts.
Diagnosis A tendency to complain, to be suspicious and to be apathetic.

Stomach (Yin Organ) (Yang Meridian)

Physiology This is a hollow organ that is largely inactive.
Damaged by Strong spice, sugar and excess salt; eating when tense or worried; overeating.
Supported by Chewing very well. Regular meals. Not eating more than two hours before sleep.
Diagnosis Being anxious, tendency to worry, a thickly coated tongue.

Lungs (Yang Organ)   (Yin Meridian)

Physiology A very active organ involved in absorption and elimination.
Damaged by Smoking; animal fats, especially eggs and meat; being unable to express your emotions easily – especially grief or sadness.
Supported by Hard green leafy vegetables, eg broccoli, watercress, dandelion leaves.
Diagnosis Pale skin, low energy. Depression.

Colon (Yin organ) (Yang meridian)

Physiology Final stage of elimination.
Damaged by Overcooked saturated animal fats, especially ham, bacon, meat pies; processed carbohydrate; holding on to the past; inability to let go of resentment.
Supported by Root vegetables, wholegrain products.
Diagnosis Flatulence, constipation, irritable bowel syndrome, swollen lower lip.

Kidney (Yang Organ) (Yin Meridian)

Physiology Designed to balance our fluid and 'electrolyte' levels (the levels of chemicals and waste in the blood).
Damaged by Ice cold fluids; excessive salt, coffee, eggs; not enough sleep; stress; damp and cold environments.
Supported by Deep sleep, keeping warm, hot fluids, pulses.
Diagnosis Tiredness, lethargy, being self-protective, dark area below the eyes.

Bladder (Yin Organ) (Yang Meridian)

Physiology Hollow inactive organ.
Damaged by Excess salt; ice cold fluid; burnt food (eg toast), coffee, chocolate; getting too tired; being exposed to the cold.
Supported by Warm foods, hot drinks, warm clothing with the lower back and midriff kept warm.
Diagnosis Damp hands, frequent urination, redness around the heel and outside of the feet.

Heart Governor (Yang Organ) (Yin Meridian)

Physiology This system governs the circulation of chi in the body which unites the inner organs. Provides energy for our libido.
Damaged by Stress; lack of sleep; too much sexual activity; lack of physical exercise to stimulate chi and blood circulation.
Supported by Having rhythm in our lives, keeping warm, having stability in our lives.
Diagnosis Irritable behaviour, heaviness in the chest, thirst.

Triple Heater (Yin Organ) (Yang Meridian)

Physiology This gathers and regulates the chi energy of the respiratory, digestive and sexual functions of the body.
Damaged by Excess cold or heat; stuffy environments.
Supported by Exercise that involves circulation (getting breathless and sweaty).
Diagnosis Feeling uncomfortable in extremes of temperature,

finding it hard to cope with the heat. Finding it very difficult to be warm when the weather is cold.

Governing Vessel (Yang System) (Yin Meridian)

Rises up the back of the body. Although not a specific organ or system, points located on this meridian are recognized to help calm the mind, bring clarity of thinking and influence our spiritual awareness.

Conception Vessel (Yin System) (Yang Meridian)

Rises centrally up the front of the body. Points found along this meridian can help with digestion, breathing and communication.

Glossary

aikido A Japanese martial art invented this century to promote flexibility and awareness.

aura An extension of the body's energy beyond the physical body.

chi Chinese word for energy, pronounced 'chee'.

chi kung A Chinese moving meditation that emphasizes the importance of breathing to promote inner strength and well-being.

cun An acupuncturist's measurement of distances between acupressure points using the patient's thumb or fingers.

dõ-in A Japanese system of self-massage based on acupressure points and meridians.

feng shui A system of holistic interior design which promotes harmony and balance between people and their environment.

fire One of the five elements transformations.

five element (transformation) theory A theory used widely in oriental medicine in which medicine is described by the elements metal, water, fire, wood/tree and earth/soil.

ki Japanese word for energy.

macrobiotics A reinvention of oriental philosophy and healing, begun this century by George Ohsawa and now taught by his students.

meridian A channel of energy on the surface of the body, relating to the internal organs. Meridians come in *pairs* – the same meridian on the left and right of the body, and *partners* – the different but equivalent meridians on the front and back of the body.

metal One of the five elements/transformations.

moxabustion The application of heat to acupressure points.

nine metal needle/plum blossom An acupuncture tool that incorporates nine small needles in a lightweight hammer head.

prana Indian word for energy.

seiza A Japanese meditation position that involves sitting on your heels with your toes under your buttocks.

shiatsu A therapy to promote healing in the body, mind and spirit by the use of pressure to the meridian system. 'Shiatsu' is a Japanese word meaning 'finger pressure'.

soil One of the five elements/transformations.

tai chi A Chinese moving meditation which emphasizes the importance of breathing and being 'centred'.

tree One of the five elements/transformations.

tsubo Acupressure point (Japanese).

water One of the five elements/transformations.

wood One of the five elements/transformations.

yin/yang The oriental concept of dynamic opposition and its being the fundamental force behind all activity and structure.

yoga A traditional Indian form of exercise stretches and meditation for enhancing relaxation, vitality and flexibility.

zen An oriental religious practice that encourages spontaneity and living in the present.

Further Reading

CLASSICAL TEXTS

These three books together give the essence of the yin/yang philosophy of change. The first two and the last introduce the principles and the third book relates these to oriental healing.

Karcher, Stephen L and Ritsema, Rudolf, *I Ching*, Element Books, UK, 1994

Lao Tzu, trans John C H Wu, *Tao Te Ching*, Shambhala, UK, 1990

Veith, Ilza, (trans), *The Yellow Emperor's Classic of Internal Medicine*, University of California Press, USA, 1966

Wilhelm, Richard (trans), *I Ching*, Routledge and Kegan Paul, UK, 1951

ACUPUNCTURE

There are many books on this subject and I particularly recommend Peter Mole's book in the same series as this one and Dr Omura's as he covers the history, the concepts, the diagnostic methods and the meridians in excellent detail.

Mole, Peter, *Acupuncture*, Element Books, UK, 1992

Omura, Dr Y, *Acupuncture Medicine*, Japan Publications, Japan, 1982

DŌ-IN

If you enjoyed the DIY routine in chapter 5, you may wish to take the subject further and develop the ideas with Kushi's book which covers many of the spiritual practices and de Langre's book which highlights dõ-in practice in other cultures also.

Kushi, Michio, *The Book of Dõ-in*, Japan Publications, Japan, 1979
de Langre, Jacques, *Dõ-in*, Happiness Press, USA, 1981

SHIATSU

A very practical way to further your interest in acupressure would be to study a complete massage system based on the meridians and acupuncture points such as shiatsu. (The Shiatsu Society can tell you more about colleges and schools that offer introductory and diploma courses – *see* Useful Addresses.)

Cowmeadow, Oliver, *The Art of Shiatsu*, Element Books, UK, 1992
Liechti, Elaine, *Shiatsu*, Element Books, UK, 1992

Useful Addresses

ACUPRESSURE

Michael Blate
Falkynor Books
PO Box 8060
Pembroke Pines
FL 33023
USA

Tony Rusli
82 Ashville Road
London E11 4DU
UK
Tel: (0)181 558 9676

Jon Sandifer
PO Box 69
Teddington
Middlesex TW11 9SH
UK
Tel: (0)973 338651

ITHMA
PO Box 6555
London N8 9DF
UK

ACUPUNCTURE

American Association of Acupuncture and Oriental Medicine
1424 16th Street NW
Suite 501
Washington DC 20036
USA

Acupuncture Ethics and Standards Organization
PO Box 84
Merrylands
NSW 2160
Australia
Tel: (02)681 4836

Council for Acupuncture
179 Gloucester Place
London NW1 6DX
UK
Tel: (0)171 724 5756

NZRA
PO Box 9950
Wellington 1
New Zealand
(04)801 64 00

DÕ-IN

The Kushi Institute
Toronto
Canada
Tel: (416) 247 0214

The Kushi Institute
Weteringschans 65
1017 RX Amsterdam
Holland
Tel: (020) 625 7513

The Kushi Institute
PO Box 7
Becket
MA 01223
USA
Tel: (413) 623 5741

SHIATSU

American Oriental Bodywork Therapy Association
50 Maple Place
Manhasset
New York 11030
USA

Japanese Shiatsu College
2–15–6 Koishikawa
Bunk Yoku
Tokyo
Japan

Shiatsu Society
31 Pullman Lane
Guildford
Surrey GU7 1XY
UK
Tel: (0)1483 860 771

Shiatsu School of Canada
547 College Street
Toronto
Canada M69 1A9
Tel: (416) 323 1818

Shiatsu Society of Ireland
Greenville Lodge
Esker Road
Lucan
Co Dublin
Eire

The Shiatsu Therapy Association of Australia
332 Carlisle Street
Balaclava
3183 Victoria
Australia

Index

Index